Diagnosis and Treatment of Thoracic Outlet Syndrome

Diagnosis and Treatment of Thoracic Outlet Syndrome

Special Issue Editors

Julie Ann Freischlag
Natalia O. Glebova

MDPI • Basel • Beijing • Wuhan • Barcelona • Belgrade

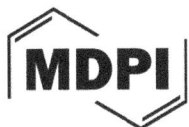

MDPI

Special Issue Editors

Julie Ann Freischlag
Wake Forest School of Medicine
USA

Natalia O. Glebova
Kaiser Permanente South Baltimore County Medical Center
USA

Editorial Office
MDPI
St. Alban-Anlage 66
Basel, Switzerland

This is a reprint of articles from the Special Issue published online in the open access journal *Diagnostics* (ISSN 2075-4418) from 2017 to 2018 (available at: http://www.mdpi.com/journal/diagnostics/special_issues/TOS)

For citation purposes, cite each article independently as indicated on the article page online and as indicated below:

LastName, A.A.; LastName, B.B.; LastName, C.C. Article Title. *Journal Name* **Year**, *Article Number, Page Range.*

ISBN 978-3-03897-025-5 (Pbk)
ISBN 978-3-03897-026-2 (PDF)

Contents

About the Special Issue Editors vii

Julie Ann Freischlag
The Art of Caring in the Treatment of Thoracic Outlet Syndrome
Reprinted from: *Diagnostics* **2018**, *8*, 35, doi: 10.3390/diagnostics8020035 1

M. Libby Weaver and Ying Wei Lum
New Diagnostic and Treatment Modalities for Neurogenic Thoracic Outlet Syndrome
Reprinted from: *Diagnostics* **2017**, *7*, 28, doi: 10.3390/diagnostics7020028 4

Meena Archie and David Rigberg
Vascular TOS—Creating a Protocol and Sticking to It
Reprinted from: *Diagnostics* **2017**, *7*, 34, doi: 10.3390/diagnostics7020034 12

Misty D. Humphries
Creating a Registry for Patients with Thoracic Outlet Syndrome
Reprinted from: *Diagnostics* **2017**, *7*, 36, doi: 10.3390/diagnostics7020036 26

David P. Kuwayama, Jason R. Lund, Charles O. Brantigan and Natalia O. Glebova
Choosing Surgery for Neurogenic TOS: The Roles of Physical Exam, Physical Therapy,
and Imaging
Reprinted from: *Diagnostics* **2017**, *7*, 37, doi: 10.3390/diagnostics7020037 31

Vanessa Leonhard, Gregory Caldwell, Mei Goh, Sean Reeder and Heather F. Smith
Ultrasonographic Diagnosis of Thoracic Outlet Syndrome Secondary to Brachial Plexus
Piercing Variation
Reprinted from: *Diagnostics* **2017**, *7*, 40, doi: 10.3390/diagnostics7030040 44

Richard J. Sanders and Stephen J. Annest
Pectoralis Minor Syndrome: Subclavicular Brachial Plexus Compression
Reprinted from: *Diagnostics* **2017**, *7*, 46, doi: 10.3390/diagnostics7030046 57

**Jesse Peek, Cornelis G. Vos, Çağdas Ünlü, Michiel A. Schreve, Rob H. W. van de Mortel and
Jean-Paul P. M. de Vries**
Long-Term Functional Outcome of Surgical Treatment for Thoracic Outlet Syndrome
Reprinted from: *Diagnostics* **2018**, *8*, 7, doi: 10.3390/diagnostics8010007 69

Colin P. Ryan, Nicolas J. Mouawad, Patrick S. Vaccaro and Michael R. Go
A Patient-Centered Approach to Guide Follow-Up and Adjunctive Testing and Treatment after
First Rib Resection for Venous Thoracic Outlet Syndrome Is Safe and Effective
Reprinted from: *Diagnostics* **2018**, *8*, 4, doi: 10.3390/diagnostics8010004 75

**Garret Adam, Kevin Wang, Christopher J. Demaree, Jenny S. Jiang, Mathew Cheung,
Carlos F. Bechara and Peter H. Lin**
A Prospective Evaluation of Duplex Ultrasound for Thoracic Outlet Syndrome in
High-Performance Musicians Playing Bowed String Instruments
Reprinted from: *Diagnostics* **2018**, *8*, 11, doi: 10.3390/diagnostics8010011 83

Sebastian Povlsen and Bo Povlsen
Diagnosing Thoracic Outlet Syndrome: Current Approaches and Future Directions
Reprinted from: *Diagnostics* **2018**, *8*, 21, doi: 10.3390/diagnostics8010021 92

About the Special Issue Editors

Julie Ann Freischlag, Professor of Surgery, CEO, Wake Forest Baptist Medical Center and Dean, Wake Forest School of Medicine. Patients with thoracic outlet syndrome present with a myriad of symptoms and treatment can range from physical therapy and pain management, to surgical intervention as well as postoperative interventions. These patients tend to be young and desire an excellent quality of life, especially if their symptoms have led to pain and discomfort preventing that lifestyle. The treatment plan will vary with each individual patient and may also vary over time. The art of taking care of these patients requires excellent listening skills and a team of specialists who can be available to manage these patients back to a life they will enjoy.

Natalia O. Glebova is a vascular surgeon in the Mid-Atlantic Permanente Medical Group. She earned an MD and a PhD at Johns Hopkins University, Medical Scientist Training Program, and a BA in Molecular Biology at the University of California, Berkeley. She completed both her general surgical training and vascular surgery fellowship at Johns Hopkins Hospital and is a Fellow of the American College of Surgeons. Her clinical interests include open surgical reconstruction and minimally invasive endovascular treatment of aortic, visceral, and peripheral artery diseases.

diagnostics

MDPI

Editorial

The Art of Caring in the Treatment of Thoracic Outlet Syndrome

Julie Ann Freischlag

Wake Forest Baptist Medical Center, Wake Forest School of Medicine, Winston-Salem, 27157 NC, USA; jfreisch@wakehealth.edu

Received: 17 April 2018; Accepted: 15 May 2018; Published: 19 May 2018

Those who diagnose and treat patients with thoracic outlet syndrome, especially those patients with neurogenic thoracic outlet syndrome, have a practice, which needs to include many modalities to diagnose, treat, and intervene to improve their quality of life for the present and for the future. Three key points constitute the mainstay of the art of caring for thoracic outlet patients. Initially, the most important thing is to make an accurate diagnosis. The second most important thing is not to offer interventions that will not help, perhaps harm, and to give false hope to those who have complex symptoms and have had interventions elsewhere without success. The third thing is to develop an algorithm of consistent evaluation and treatment for each patient to ensure an optimal outcome.

Maintaining a registry of your patients to truly understand your results and failures is essential. It is only by recognizing how your patients have done over time do you learn how best to take care of the next patient who seeks your help. We have learned that those neurogenic patients who are over the age of 40, and have had a dependency on narcotics for a long period of time, have other issues such as cervical disc disease, shoulder issues, and have a negative scalene block do not do as well with surgical intervention [1,2]. Additionally, those who undergo first rib resection and anterior scalenectomy, and never improve, usually fail to improve with a second operation. Whereas those who initially improve and then have recurrent symptoms about a year later with or without a history of repeat injury, can be treated with physical therapy and or Botox injections with great success [3]. Additionally, we know that about 50% of patients who have undergone first rib resection and anterior scalenectomy for venous thrombosis will have significant residual stenosis, which requires intervention to prevent recurrent thrombosis [4].

These 10 monographs offer the following salient points to improve your care of the patient with thoracic outlet syndrome:

Weaver and Lum summarize the new diagnostic and treatment modalities for those patients with neurogenic thoracic outlet syndrome [5]. They review the imaging techniques of computed tomography (CT) and magnetic resonance imaging (MRI) along with the value of median antebrachial cutaneous nerve (MABC) sensory nerve action potentials in identifying impingement if the brachial plexus. Updates in surgical techniques are reviewed including robotic and endoscopic approaches.

The importance of selecting a protocol in the treatment of vascular thoracic outlet syndrome is discussed by Archie and Rigberg [6]. They described their protocols in the treatment of both venous and arterial thoracic outlet syndrome. The treatment of both acute and chronic venous thrombosis, along with acute thrombosis, claudication, and asymptomatic arterial presentations, are delineated with excellent case report examples.

Humphries outlines the scope of a thoracic outlet syndrome registry and points out the important data to collect [7]. She also described how the combination of multiple registries in the future can play a role in the treatment of a condition like thoracic outlet syndrome due to the fact that many practitioners do not see a large number of patients.

Choosing the correct treatment, the correct timing of the treatment, and the succession to a different treatment for the patient with neurogenic thoracic outlet syndrome is the key for long-term success in alleviating symptoms for these patients [8]. These authors emphasize the need for a complete history and physical exam which will lead to the right intervention. They also outline the mainstay of the appropriate physical therapy protocol and the use of anterior scalene blocks.

The use of ultrasound in identifying anatomic variants in patients with thoracic outlet are described in detail by Leonhard and colleagues [9]. Utilizing both cadaver necks (82) and student subjects (22), brachial plexus variation was seen in 62.1% and 21%, respectively. Of the students, 50% had neurogenic thoracic outlet symptoms, which was higher than those with classic anatomy (14%). Ultrasonography can be helpful in diagnosis of neurogenic thoracic outlet syndrome, especially if provocative testing is negative.

The diagnosis and treatment of pectoralis minor syndrome is discussed in detail by Sanders and Annest [10]. This anatomical variant of thoracic outlet syndrome is rare but can be differentiated from neurogenic thoracic outlet syndrome by symptoms and physical exam, especially tenderness found in the axillary area. A pectoralis minor block can be used similarly to an anterior scalene block to make the diagnosis.

Utilizing a patient-centered care appraisal regarding symptoms before and after first rib resection, Ryan and colleagues tailor their diagnostic tests and intervention in patients with venous compression (McCleary's syndrome) or venous thrombosis [11]. Their findings in 59 patients, who underwent first rib resection and anterior scalenectomy, demonstrated no difference in outcome if the patient had received thrombolysis, or when the rib resection had been performed which matched similar findings by Guzzo and colleagues [12]. Their conclusion is that paying attention to patient symptoms and not just vein patency can lead to appropriate intervention in patients with venous thoracic outlet syndrome.

Peek and colleagues report on a retrospective multicenter study on patients who underwent operations for thoracic outlet syndrome from 2005 to 2016 [13]. Patients were assessed by the 11 item version of the QuickDASH questionnaire. Sixty-two patients were evaluated—36 neurogenic, 13 arterial, 7 venous, and 6 combined—and 73% returned the survey. Fifty-four percent (27) had complete relief and 90% had improvement. These findings were similar to previous findings by Chang [14] and Rochlin [15], when patients are chosen appropriately.

A unique report on high performance musicians who played bowed string instruments is presented by Adam and colleagues [16]. Sixty-four high performance musicians were evaluated and compared to 52 healthy volunteers with duplex scanning and provocative maneuvers. Duplex scans were abnormal in 69% of musicians showing compression, as compared to 15% of controls ($p = 0.03$), and provocative maneuvers were positive in 44% of musicians as compared to 3% of controls ($p = 0.03$). This alerts us to the high incidence of potential thoracic outlet syndrome in these musicians as many of us has seen and treated them.

An excellent summary of the present state of the art of diagnosis, treatment, and outcomes is presented by Povlsen and Polvsen [17]. They hypothesize that the ability to stratify patients according to their exact compressive mechanism could lead to better outcomes.

In summary, these 10 informative manuscripts provide a roadmap for the future excellent treatment of those patients with thoracic outlet syndrome.

Conflicts of Interest: The author declare no conflict of interest.

References

1. Orlando, M.S.; Likes, K.C.; Mirza, S.; Cao, Y.; Cohen, A.; Lum, Y.W.; Reifsnyder, T.; Freischlag, J.A. A decade of excellent outcomes after surgical intervention in 538 patients with thoracic outlet syndrome. *J. Am. Coll. Surg.* **2015**, *220*, 934–939. [CrossRef] [PubMed]
2. Lum, Y.W.; Brooke, B.S.; Likes, K.; Modi, M.; Grunebach, H.; Christo, P.J.; Freischlag, J.A. Impact of anterior scalenectomy blocks on predicting surgical success in older patients with neurogenic thoracic outlet syndrome. *J. Vasc. Surg.* **2012**, *55*, 1370–1375. [CrossRef] [PubMed]

3. Likes, K.C.; Orlando, M.S.; Salditch, Q.; Mirza, S.; Cohen, A.; Reifsnyder, T.; Lum, Y.W.; Freischlag, J.A. Lessons Learned in the Surgical Treatment of Neurogenic Thoracic Outlet Syndrome over 10 Years. *Vasc. Endovasc. Surg.* **2015**, *49*, 8–11. [CrossRef] [PubMed]

4. DeLeon, R.A.; Chang, D.C.; Hassoun, H.T.; Black, J.H.; Roseborough, G.S.; Perler, B.A.; Rotellini-Coltvet, L.; Call, D.; Busse, C.; Freischlag, J.A. Multiple treatment algorithms for successful outcomes in venous thoracic outlet syndrome. *Surgery* **2009**, *145*, 500–507. [CrossRef] [PubMed]

5. Weaver, M.L.; Lum, Y.W. New diagnostic and treatment modalities for neurogenic thoracic outlet syndrome. *Diagnostics* **2017**, *7*, 28. [CrossRef] [PubMed]

6. Archie, A.; Rigberg, D. Vascular TOS-creating a protocol and sticking to it. *Diagnostics* **2017**, *7*, 34. [CrossRef] [PubMed]

7. Humphries, M.D. Creating a registry for patients with thoracic outlet syndrome. *Diagnostics* **2017**, *7*, 36. [CrossRef] [PubMed]

8. Kuwayama, D.P.; Lund, J.R.; Brantigan, C.O.; Glebova, N.O. Choosing surgery for neurogenic TOS: The roles of physical exam, physical therapy and imaging. *Diagnostics* **2017**, *7*, 37. [CrossRef] [PubMed]

9. Leonhard, V.; Caldwell, G.; Goh, M.; Reeder, S.; Smith, H.F. Ultrasonographic diagnosis of thoracic outlet syndrome secondary to brachial plexus piercing variation. *Diagnostics* **2017**, *7*, 40. [CrossRef] [PubMed]

10. Sanders, R.J.; Annest, S.J. Pectoralis minor syndrome: Subclavicular brachial plexus compression. *Diagnostics* **2017**, *7*, 46. [CrossRef] [PubMed]

11. Ryan, C.P.; Mouawad, N.J.; Vaccaro, P.S.; Go, M.R. A patient-centered approach to guide follow-up and adjunctive testing and treatment after first rib resection for venous thoracic outlet syndrome is safe and effective. *Diagnostics* **2018**, *8*, 4. [CrossRef] [PubMed]

12. Guzzo, J.L.; Chang, K.; Demos, J.; Black, J.H.; Freischlag, J.A. Preoperative thrombolysis and venoplasty affords no benefit in patency following first rib resection and scalenectomy for subacute and chronic subclavian vein thrombosis. *J. Vasc. Surg.* **2010**, *52*, 658–662. [CrossRef] [PubMed]

13. Peek, J.; Vos, C.G.; Unlu, C.; Schreve, M.A.; van de Mortel, R.H.W.; de Vries, J.-P. Long-term functional outcome of surgical treatment for thoracic outlet syndrome. *Diagnostics* **2018**, *8*, 7. [CrossRef] [PubMed]

14. Chang, D.C.; Rotellini-Coltvet, L.A.; Mukherjeed, D.; DeLeon, R.; Freischlag, J.A. Surgical intervention for thoracic outlet syndrome improves patient's quality of life. *J. Vasc. Surg.* **2009**, *49*, 630–637. [CrossRef] [PubMed]

15. Rochlin, D.H.; Gilson, M.M.; Likes, K.C.; Graf, E.; Ford, N.; Christo, P.J.; Freischlag, J.A. Quality-of-life scores in neurogenic thoracic outlet syndrome patients undergoing first rib resection and scalenectomy. *J. Vasc. Surg.* **2013**, *57*, 436–443. [CrossRef] [PubMed]

16. Adam, G.; Wang, K.; Demaree, C.J.; Jiang, J.S.; Cheung, M.; Bechara, C.F.; Lin, P.H. A prospective evaluation of duplex ultrasound for thoracic outlet syndrome in high-performance musicians playing bowed string instruments. *Diagnostics* **2018**, *8*, 11. [CrossRef] [PubMed]

17. Povlsen, S.; Polvsen, B. Diagnosing thoracic outlet syndrome: Current approaches and future directions. *Diagnostics* **2018**, *8*, 21. [CrossRef] [PubMed]

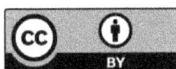

diagnostics

MDPI

Review

New Diagnostic and Treatment Modalities for Neurogenic Thoracic Outlet Syndrome

M. Libby Weaver[1] and Ying Wei Lum[2,*]

[1] Department of Surgery, Johns Hopkins Hospital, Baltimore, MD 21287, USA; weave25@jhmi.edu
[2] Department of Surgery, Johns Hopkins Heart and Vascular Institute, Johns Hopkins Medical Centers, Baltimore, MD 21287, USA
* Correspondence: ylum1@jhmi.edu; Tel.: +1-410-955-5165

Academic Editor: Andreas Kjaer
Received: 1 March 2017; Accepted: 24 May 2017; Published: 27 May 2017

Abstract: Neurogenic thoracic outlet syndrome is a widely recognized, yet controversial, syndrome. The lack of specific objective diagnostic modalities makes diagnosis difficult. This is compounded by a lack of agreed upon definitive criteria to confirm diagnosis. Recent efforts have been made to more clearly define a set of diagnostic criteria that will bring consistency to the diagnosis of neurogenic thoracic syndrome. Additionally, advancements have been made in the quality and techniques of various imaging modalities that may aid in providing more accurate diagnoses. Surgical decompression remains the mainstay of operative treatment; and minimally invasive techniques are currently in development to further minimize the risks of this procedure. Medical management continues to be refined to provide non-operative treatment modalities for certain patients, as well. The aim of the present work is to review these updates in the diagnosis and treatment of neurogenic thoracic outlet syndrome.

Keywords: neurogenic thoracic outlet syndrome; brachial plexus compression; brachial plexopathy

1. Introduction

Neurogenic Thoracic Outlet Syndrome (nTOS) is a clinical diagnosis that describes the symptomatic manifestation of the compression of the neurologic structures traversing the thoracic outlet, namely the brachial plexus. It is the most common of the three subtypes of TOS representing 95% of overall TOS occurrences, with women aged 20–40 being the primary population affected, yet it is the most controversial for several reasons [1,2]. With nTOS, unlike arterial and venous TOS, diagnosis is largely clinical and subjective in nature, with no definitive imaging or diagnostic studies available to confirm its presence. Until recently, there were no clear guidelines to define specifically which patients clearly demonstrate a clinical diagnosis of nTOS. New developments in objective diagnostic studies, as well as more clearly-defined guidelines for proper diagnosis of nTOS help to better identify patients suffering from nTOS so that these patients may receive appropriate treatment. Therapeutic modalities for nTOS range from medical to operative in nature. Several surgical approaches, including supra-clavicular and trans-axillary, are utilized with equivalent rates of success. However, new surgical approaches, including video-assisted thoracoscopic, endoscopic-assisted and robotic approaches also demonstrate excellent outcomes.

2. Diagnostic Criteria

Until recently, a vital challenge in the efficient and adequate treatment of patients suffering from nTOS was the lack of agreed upon diagnostic criteria. The Consortium for Outcomes Research and Education of Thoracic Outlet Syndrome recently developed a preliminary set of diagnostic criteria for nTOS. This group consists of physicians and scientists from multiple disciplines working together with the intention of assisting practitioners in accurately identifying, and thus employing appropriate management strategies for, those patients presenting with symptoms suggestive of nTOS. These guidelines clearly delineate combinations of history and physical examination findings that are required to properly diagnose, and thus treat, nTOS, as outlined in Table 1. The findings must be present for a minimum of three months and must not be attributable to any other neurologic cause [3].

Table 1. Preliminary criteria for the clinical diagnosis of Neurogenic Thoracic Outlet Syndrome (nTOS).

Unilateral or Bilateral Upper Extremity Symptoms	
(1) Extend beyond the distribution of a single cervical nerve root or peripheral nerve (2) Have been present for at least 12 weeks (3) Have not been satisfactorily explained by another condition (4) Meet at least one criterion in at least four of the following five categories:	
1. Principal Symptoms	1A. Pain in the neck, upper back, shoulder, arm and/or hand 1B. Numbness, paresthesias and/or weakness in the arm, hand or digits
2. Symptom Characteristics	2A. Pain/paresthesias/weakness exacerbated with elevated arm positions 2B. Pain/paresthesias/weakness exacerbated with prolonged or repetitive arm/hand use or by prolonged work on a keyboard or other repetitive strain 2C. Pain/paresthesias radiate down the arm from the supraclavicular or infraclavicular space
3. Clinical History	3A. Symptoms began after occupational, recreational or accidental injury of the head, neck or upper extremity, including repetitive upper extremity strain or overuse activity 3B. Previous clavicle or first rib fracture or known cervical rib(s) 3C. Previous cervical spine or peripheral nerve surgery without sustained improvement 3D. Previous conservative or surgical treatment for TOS
4. Physical Examination	4A. Local tenderness on palpation over scalene triangle or subcoracoid space 4B. Arm/hand/digit paresthesias on palpation over scalene triangle or subcoracoid space 4C. Weak handgrip, intrinsic muscles, or Digit 5, or thenar/hypothenar atrophy
5. Provocative Maneuvers	5A. Positive Upper Limb Tension Test (ULTT) 5B. Positive 1- or 3-min Elevated Arm Stress Test (EAST)

Additionally, the Society for Vascular Surgery published reporting standards for TOS, the primary aim of which is to provide a clear and consistent understanding and definition of what constitutes a diagnosis of nTOS, while also accurately assessing the results of various management strategies. This more simplistic definition consists of the following four criteria: signs and symptoms of pathology occurring at the thoracic outlet (pain and/or tenderness), signs and symptoms of nerve compression (distal neurologic changes, often worse with arms overhead or dangling), absence of other pathology potentially explaining the symptoms and a positive response to a properly-performed scalene muscle test injection [4]. The subjective nature of many of these diagnostic findings contributes to the controversy surrounding the validity of the diagnosis of nTOS.

3. Diagnostic Techniques

3.1. Imaging

There are objective radiologic diagnostic findings in some, but not all, patients who fit the criteria for diagnosis of nTOS. Although imaging modalities, particularly ultrasonography, are generally able to provide conclusive evidence of the presence of vascular forms of TOS, the efficacy of diagnostic imaging modalities in the evaluation of nTOS is less clear. Nonetheless, imaging may prove to be a useful adjunct in the diagnosis of nTOS. Ultrasonography, for example, may demonstrate associated vascular compression in those patients presenting with symptoms suggestive of nTOS. In one study of 143 patients with nTOS symptoms, duplex scanning demonstrated ipsilateral compression of vessels in 31% of these patients, compared to only 8% demonstrating asymptomatic contralateral compression and 10% bilateral compression when patients' arms were placed in abducted positioning [5]. These results suggest that findings of vascular compression may be present even in nTOS, providing additional support of the diagnosis. Ultrasonography may also demonstrate signs specific to nTOS. One study describes the "wedge-sickle sign", identification of a fibromuscular structure causing indentation of the lower trunk of the brachial plexus. The structure itself is hyper-echoic in nature, while the lower trunk is hypo-echoic due to loss of the nerve fascicle. In this study, the presence of the wedge-sickle sign was highly sensitive (95%) with a positive predictive value of 82.6% [6].

Computed Tomography (CT) and Magnetic Resonance Imaging (MRI) may be utilized to assess for compression of the brachial plexus as it traverses the thoracic outlet. They can identify bony abnormalities or fibromuscular abnormalities and anatomic variants which may predispose patients to the development of nTOS. Specifically, these imaging studies can identify abnormal branching patterns or an abnormal course of the brachial plexus, each of which may be associated with nerve compression. Dynamic changes causing narrowing of those spaces through which the brachial plexus traverses may also predispose patients to nTOS and may be identifiable with proper positioning of the patient when obtaining images [3]. The utility of MRI appears to be dependent on the specific technique utilized. One study examined 42 cases of TOS, which were managed with surgical decompression. This study demonstrated poor correlation between MRI and intraoperative findings. The sensitivity and specificity of MRI for diagnosis of TOS in this study was 41% and 33%, respectively [7]. Alternatively, MR Neurography (MRN) shows potential as a beneficial diagnostic tool for nTOS [8]. Specifically, variations of MRN such as Short Tau Inversion Recovery (STIR) sequences and the Spectral Adiabatic Inversion Recovery (SPAIR) preparatory module deliver a more complete anatomical description of the nerves comprising the brachial plexus. Additionally, the use of diffusion tensor imaging sequences to visualize nerve fascicles is employed in the modeling technique of tractography, which allows for a more comprehensive assessment of peripheral nerve injury [9]. One study using MRN demonstrated a 100% positive predictive value in all thirty patients. In this study, however, compression was also identifiable using ultrasonography in all patients with MRN-identified nerve lesions [10].

Electrodiagnostic testing is also of utility in the diagnosis of nTOS. These tests can serve to rule out other neurologic etiologies as contributors to a patient's symptomatology. In addition, axonal loss of brachial plexus neurons is present on electrodiagnostic testing in those patients ultimately diagnosed with nTOS. When comparing the Median Antebrachial Cutaneous Nerve (MABC), which arises from T1 nerve fibers, to sensory nerve fibers derived from the level of C8, nerve conduction of the MABC demonstrates abnormal amplitudes. Thus, combined evaluation of nerve fibers originating at both levels is recommended [11]. When evaluating nTOS, several studies over the last decade suggest that the most sensitive diagnostic nerve conduction study is the demonstration of a diminished amplitude in MABC Sensory Nerve Action Potential (SNAP). One study in particular revealed abnormal MABC SNAP in 85.7% of patients diagnosed with nTOS compared to ulnar SNAP (77.8%) and median and ulnar compound muscle action potentials (55.6% and 33.3%, respectively) [12]. Still, reduced SNAP of the ulnar nerve or decreased thenar M-wave voltage are associated with impingement of the brachial plexus [3].

3.2. Scalene Injection

Another diagnostic modality that is important in the evaluation of nTOS is scalene injection. Although this technique is not new, it continues to undergo modifications that further enhance its diagnostic efficacy. Scalene injection can be a qualitative diagnostic tool that is additionally predictive of surgical outcomes in those patients under consideration for surgical management. It may also be considered as an alternative treatment modality for appropriately selected patients. In one study, work performance, power and time to fatigue were measured on patients undergoing anterior scalene muscle block with 1% lidocaine injection during a variety of exercises following the procedure. The results demonstrated statistically-significant increases in function motor capacity. This suggests that anterior scalene muscle blocks may provide quantifiable information that may assist in successful and accurate diagnosis of nTOS [13]. High-performance athletes are a special population that may require a more intense post-procedural exercise regimen to accurately assess the effect on patient symptomatology and verify a successful scalene block [14].

Further refining the diagnostic techniques outlined above, as well as developing new objective diagnostic tools, is important not only to improve accuracy and consistency in the diagnosis of nTOS, but also to allow for the diagnosis to be made in a more efficient and timely manner. In nTOS in particular, early surgical intervention following symptom onset is associated with improved patient outcomes, particularly in patients greater than forty years of age [15,16]. The utility of clinical presentation in the diagnosis of TOS, however, remains extremely important, and its value cannot be overemphasized. A retrospective review of 621 patients at one institution who were either self-referred of referred by another physician to vascular surgeons for suspicion of TOS demonstrated high diagnostic accuracy by both referring physicians and patients themselves, with 91% and 97% respectively ultimately being diagnosed with TOS [17]. This underscores the significance of recognizing clinical characteristics consistent with TOS to establish the proper diagnosis.

3.3. Genetics

Finally, it is worthwhile to mention the role of genetics in the diagnosis of TOS. Although no specific genetic mutations have been identified in association with the development of TOS, there is at least one case report of TOS presenting in multiple family members, suggesting the potential for a genetic predisposition to development of the syndrome [18]. In particular, variations in HOX gene expression are implicated in the development of anomalies of the axial skeleton, including the presence of a cervical first rib [19]. With the increasing use of genetics in medicine, it is possible that genetic analysis will become an important factor in the diagnosis of TOS in the future.

4. Treatment

4.1. Surgical Management

4.1.1. Patient Selection and Surgical Outcomes

With proper patient selection, the operative management of nTOS has excellent outcomes. Appropriate patient selection and management is a key determining factor in surgical success. Successful stratification of patients into appropriate management protocols is accomplished with implementation of several selection strategies. Exclusion of cervical or other peripheral nerve compression syndromes is a critical component of a thorough preoperative evaluation. Patients who are less than 40 years of age, present with a shorter symptoms duration and are non-smokers have better outcomes than other patients undergoing surgical management of TOS [20,21]. One vascular surgery referral center determined only 1/3 of the 621 patients referred for surgical intervention were appropriate candidates for First Rib Resection with Scalenectomy (FRRS). This institution demonstrated a 91% surgical success rate in those who were offered operative management [20]. This institute selects patients with nTOS who are refractory to an eight-week course of physical therapy and responsive to anterior scalene muscle blocks with Botox or lidocaine for surgical intervention [1]. In contrast, another major referral center for TOS implements an approach in which nTOS patients are deemed appropriate for operative management only if they demonstrate symptomatic improvement with 8–16 weeks of physical therapy. One study from this institution reports 24 of 59 patients referred for further evaluation of nTOS were candidates for surgical intervention with a comparable rate of symptomatic improvement in 90% at one year [22]. There is evidence, however, that a subset of patients presenting with nTOS with co-existing arterial involvement is refractory to, and sometimes worsened with, physical therapy. Ultimately, these patients demonstrate even better outcomes than those with nTOS only after surgical intervention, with 100% showing improvement or resolution of neurogenic symptoms post-operatively in one study [23].

Anterior scalene blocks with lidocaine may be used to predict patients who will respond positively to operative intervention, particularly in patients over the age of forty. In this patient population, those who had a successful response to scalene blocks demonstrated an 81% success rate after surgery as compared to only a 67% surgical success rate in those patients who failed to respond to a scalene block pre-operatively. Response to scalene block was not as predictive of surgical success in patients under the age of 40 in this study. Additionally, patients over the age of 40 who presented with a longer duration of symptoms had a significantly lower rate of positive surgical outcomes. Patients less than forty years of age did not demonstrate this association [16]. These findings reiterate the importance of appropriate patient selection when evaluating those patients over the age of 40 for surgical management.

Assessment of the vascular structures of the thoracic outlet may also be an important component of the pre-operative evaluation of patients presenting with nTOS. Even without vascular symptoms, internal jugular and subclavian vein stenoses have a high incidence in patients presenting with nTOS. One study revealed stenosis of >66% within these vessels in up to 68% of these patients [24]. Although it is unclear what relationship this finding may have with surgical outcomes, recognition of asymptomatic vascular changes in patients presenting with neurogenic TOS symptoms may be useful information when determining patient appropriateness for surgical intervention.

4.1.2. Updates in Surgical Techniques

Traditionally, surgical management of nTOS consists of scalenectomy alone versus scalenectomy in combination with resection of the first rib and/or cervical rib when applicable. Various approaches including supraclavicular, infraclavicular and transaxillary approaches are all employed with equivalent excellent outcomes achieved at high volume centers. The authors' institution primarily utilizes the transaxillary approach for nTOS and reports a greater than 90% rate of improvement, or full resolution, of symptoms in 308 patients undergoing first rib resection and scalenectomy [20].

Although the transaxillary approach requires only a single small incision that is discretely placed in the axilla, other "minimally-invasive" approaches have been developed in recent years. Some institutions describe the use of Video-Assisted Thoracoscopic Surgery (VATS) as a minimally-invasive approach to first rib resection, with one reported advantage of this approach being a clearer visualization of the operative field, potentially minimizing injury to the neurovascular bundle. One institute utilizes a three-incision method in which two working and one scope port are placed. Although their data include a very small group of 10 patients, they did observe complete resolution of symptoms in 90% of patients, which is comparable to the success rate of other techniques. The median operative time was 85 min, and the median post-operative length of stay was 72 h [25]. A larger study examined 58 patients undergoing 66 rib resections (eight bilateral) with a different VATS technique requiring a transaxillary incision with a single port placement just below the incision. With this technique, 88.7% had resolution of headaches, although outcomes associated with other neurologic symptoms are unclear. Post-operative complications developed in 12% of the patients. These complications included surgical site infection, pneumothorax, pulmonary embolism and pneumonia. The average length of hospital stay post-operatively was 2.5 days [26].

Another minimally-invasive technique described in the literature is that of robotic first rib resection. One institution reports excellent results in five patients who underwent robotic first rib resection for venous TOS with no reported morbidities. This technique requires four incisions in total. At one-year follow-up, all patients maintained patent subclavian veins without any additional intervention. The average length of hospital stay was three days [27]. A later series from this institution evaluated the outcomes of robotic first rib resection for venous TOS in 13 patients and continued to demonstrate similar results with 100% vein patency at six months and a mean post-operative hospital stay of three days. The mean operative time in this study was 163 ± 39 min, which is longer than the average operative time of the other previously-established surgical approaches [28]. Given that most experienced centers routinely performing first rib resection with traditional approaches via the supraclavicular or transaxillary incision have a much shorter length of hospital stay of one day post-operatively and that these approaches require only a single incision, implementation of the above techniques has not yet occurred on a large scale [1].

A final novel technique that is worth mentioning is that of the endoscopic-assisted transaxillary approach. This approach aims to decrease the risk of pneumothoraces, a complication that is observed at a rate of 10–23% of patients undergoing transaxillary first rib resection [1,29]. One series of 22 patients undergoing first rib resection with the endoscopic-assisted transaxillary approach for better visualization of the operative field reported no complications associated with vascular, neural or pleural damage with success rates comparable to those of the traditional transaxillary approach [30].

Surgical complications associated with decompression of the thoracic outlet include pneumothorax, wound infection, hematoma and hemothorax. At our institution, there were no arterial, venous or nerve root injuries in ten years of treating 538 patients undergoing 594 FRRS procedures, 308 of which were for the neurogenic form of TOS specifically [20]. It should also be noted that there is evidence that surgical outcomes in those patients presenting with work-associated injuries and with workers' compensation are worse. One study demonstrates 60% of patients remained disabled and unable to continue work-required activities at one year after surgical intervention [31].

4.2. Medical Management

Despite the high rate of success with minimal complications associated with surgical decompression, medical management may be the most appropriate option for certain patients. These measures are effective in up to 70% of patients presenting with nTOS. Physical therapy, modifications to daily activities to keep symptom exacerbation at a minimum and complementation of the treatment regimen with pharmacologic agents are all medical measures that may be employed in the treatment of nTOS [32]. Up to 1/3 of athletes presenting with nTOS return to full function with physical therapy alone. Duration to symptom onset may be associated with increased success of medical management, as patients in this study experienced a short duration of symptoms with a mean of three months from symptom onset to evaluation and intervention [33].

Anterior scalene muscle injection not only serves as a both diagnostic and prognostic tool; it also plays a role as a therapeutic tool in patients with nTOS. A recent study shows 88.2% of 142 patients treated with scalene injections of Marcaine and triamcinolone demonstrated symptomatic improvement or resolution. Shorter symptom duration prior to the first injection was associated with increased improvement in those patients with a traumatic etiology, while the response of patients presenting with other etiologies of TOS was not affected by symptom duration [34]. Alternatively, a double-blind, randomized, controlled trial of 38 subjects did not demonstrate significant improvement in pain in patients undergoing anterior scalene injection with Botox vs. placebo. Notably, patients enrolled in this study had a mean symptom duration of six years [35].

5. Summary

In conclusion, neurogenic thoracic outlet syndrome remains a challenging entity to diagnose, but demonstrates excellent outcomes once a diagnosis is confirmed and treatment initiated. Recent statements clarify the defining factors of neurogenic thoracic outlet syndrome by clearly outlining a set of criteria consistent with the diagnosis of nTOS. The development of a clear set of criteria for diagnosis will allow for further advancements in the diagnosis and management of nTOS. Imaging studies continue to evolve as new modalities with higher quality allow for the possibility of the development of objective measures for the diagnosis of nTOS. First rib resection with anterior scalenectomy remains the operation of choice for decompression, but surgical advancements continue with the use of minimally-invasive approaches. Refinement of medical management strategies continues to offer additional non-operative treatment modalities to those patients who do not prove to be good candidates for surgical intervention or who prefer not to undergo surgical intervention.

Conflicts of Interest: The authors declare no conflict of interest.

References

1. Orlando, M.S.; Likes, K.C.; Mirza, S.; Cao, Y.; Cohen, A.; Lum, Y.W.; Reifsnyder, T.; Freischlag, J.A. A decade of excellent outcomes after surgical intervention in 538 patients with thoracic outlet syndrome. *J. Am. Coll. Surg.* **2015**, *220*, 934–939. [CrossRef] [PubMed]
2. Moore, R.; Lum, Y.W. Venous thoracic outlet syndrome. *Vasc. Med.* **2015**, *20*, 182–189. [CrossRef] [PubMed]
3. Illig, K.A. *Thoracic Outlet Syndrome*; Thompson, R.W., Freischlag, J.A., Eds.; Springer Science and Business Media: New York, NY, USA, 2014.
4. Illig, K.A.; Donohue, D.; Duncan, A.; Freischlag, J.; Gelabert, H.; Johansen, K.; Jordan, S.; Sanders, R.; Thompson, R. Reporting standards of the Society for Vascular Surgery for thoracic outlet syndrome. *J. Vasc. Surg.* **2016**, *64*, e23–e35. [CrossRef] [PubMed]
5. Orlando, M.S.; Likes, K.C.; Mirza, S.; Cao, Y.; Cohen, A.; Lum, Y.W.; Julie, A.; Freischlag, J.A. Preoperative Duplex Scanning is a Helpful Diagnostic Tool in Neurogenic Thoracic Outlet Syndrome. *Vasc. Endovasc. Surg.* **2016**, *50*, 29–32. [CrossRef] [PubMed]
6. Aranyi, Z.; Csillik, A.; Bohm, J.; Schelle, T. Ultrasonographic Identification of Fibromuscular Bands Associated with Neurogenic Thoracic Outlet Syndrome: The "Wedge-Sickle" Sign. *Ultrasound Med. Biol.* **2016**, *42*, 2357–2366. [CrossRef] [PubMed]
7. Singh, V.K.; Jeyaseelan, L.; Kyriacou, S.; Ghosh, S.; Sinisi, M.; Fox, M. Diagnostic value of magnetic resonance imaging in thoracic outlet syndrome. *J. Orthop. Surg.* **2014**, *22*, 228–231. [CrossRef] [PubMed]
8. Cejas, C.; Rollan, C.; Michelin, G.; Nogues, M. High resolution neurography of the brachial plexus by 3 Tesla magnetic resonance imaging. *Radiologia* **2016**, *58*, 88–100. [CrossRef] [PubMed]
9. Magill, S.T.; Brus-Ramer, M.; Weinstein, P.R.; Chin, C.T.; Jacques, L. Neurogenic thoracic outlet syndrome: current diagnostic criteria and advances in MRI diagnostics. *Neurosurg. Focus* **2015**, *39*, 1–5. [CrossRef] [PubMed]
10. Baumer, P.; Kele, H.; Kretschmer, T.; Koenig, R.; Pedro, M.; Bendszus, M.; Pham, M. Thoracic outlet syndrome in 3T MR neurography-Fibrous bands causing discernible lesions of the lower brachial plexus. *Eur. Radiol.* **2014**, *24*, 756–761. [CrossRef] [PubMed]
11. Tsao, B.E.; Ferrante, M.A.; Wilbourn, A.J.; Shields, R.W. Electrodiagnostic features of true neurogenic thoracic outlet syndrome. *Muscle Nerve* **2014**, *49*, 724–727. [CrossRef] [PubMed]
12. Ko, K.; Sung, D.H.; Kang, M.J.; Ko, M.J.; Do, J.G.; Sunwoo, H.; Kwon, T.G.; Hwang, J.M.; Park, Y. Clinical, Electrophysiological Findings in Adult Patients with Non-traumatic Plexopathies. *Ann. Rehabil. Med.* **2011**, *35*, 807. [CrossRef] [PubMed]
13. Braun, R.M.; Shah, K.N.; Rechnic, M.; Doehr, S.; Woods, N. Quantitative assessment of scalene muscle block for the diagnosis of suspected thoracic outlet syndrome. *J. Hand Surg. Am.* **2015**, *40*, 2255–2261. [CrossRef] [PubMed]
14. Bottros, M.M.; AuBuchon, J.D.; McLaughlin, L.N.; Altchek, D.W.; Illig, K.A.; Thompson, R.W. Exercise-Enhanced, Ultrasound-Guided Anterior Scalene Muscle/Pectoralis Minor Muscle Blocks Can Facilitate the Diagnosis of Neurogenic Thoracic Outlet Syndrome in the High-Performance Overhead Athlete. *Am. J. Sports Med.* **2017**. [CrossRef] [PubMed]
15. Al-Hashel, J.Y.; El Shorbgy, A.A.M.A.; Ahmed, S.F.; Elshereef, R.R. Early versus Late Surgical Treatment for Neurogenic Thoracic Outlet Syndrome. *ISRN Neurol.* **2013**, *2013*, 673020. [CrossRef] [PubMed]
16. Lum, Y.W.; Brooke, B.S.; Likes, K.; Modi, M.; Grunebach, H.; Christo, P.J.; Freischlag, J.A. Impact of anterior scalene lidocaine blocks on predicting surgical success in older patients with neurogenic thoracic outlet syndrome. *J. Vasc. Surg.* **2012**, *55*, 1370–1375. [CrossRef] [PubMed]
17. Likes, K.; Rochlin, D.H.; Salditch, Q.; Dapash, T.; Baker, Y.; Deguzman, R.; Selvarajah, S.; Freischlag, J.A. Diagnostic accuracy of physician and self-referred patients for thoracic outlet syndrome is excellent. *Ann. Vasc. Surg.* **2014**, *28*, 1100–1105. [CrossRef] [PubMed]

18. Janák, D.; Novotný, K.; Roček, M.; Rohn, V. Thoracic Outlet Syndrome: A Significant Family Genetic Phenotypic Presentation. *Prague Med. Rep.* **2016**, *117*, 117–123. [CrossRef] [PubMed]
19. Bots, J.; Wijnaendts, L.C.D.; Delen, S.; van Dongen, S.; Heikinheimo, K.; Galis, F. Analysis of cervical ribs in a series of human fetuses. *J. Anat.* **2011**, *219*, 403–409. [CrossRef] [PubMed]
20. Likes, K.C.; Orlando, M.S.; Salditch, Q.; Mirza, S.; Cohen, A.; Reifsnyder, T.; Lum, Y.W.; Freischlag, J.A. Lessons Learned in the Surgical Treatment of Neurogenic Thoracic Outlet Syndrome over 10 Years. *Vasc. Endovasc. Surg.* **2015**, *49*, 8–11. [CrossRef] [PubMed]
21. Rochlin, D.H.; Orlando, M.S.; Likes, K.C.; Jacobs, C.; Freischlag, J.A. Bilateral first rib resection and scalenectomy is effective for treatment of thoracic outlet syndrome. *J. Vasc. Surg.* **2014**, *60*, 185–190. [CrossRef] [PubMed]
22. Chandra, V.; Olcott, C.; Lee, J.T. Early results of a highly selective algorithm for surgery on patients with neurogenic thoracic outlet syndrome. *J. Vasc. Surg.* **2011**, *54*, 1698–1705. [CrossRef] [PubMed]
23. Likes, K.; Rochlin, D.H.; Call, D.; Freischlag, J.A. Coexistence of arterial compression in patients with neurogenic thoracic outlet syndrome. *JAMA Surg.* **2014**, *149*, 1240–1243. [CrossRef] [PubMed]
24. Ahn, S.S.; Miller, T.J.; Chen, S.W.; Chen, J.F. Internal jugular vein stenosis is common in patients presenting with neurogenic thoracic outlet syndrome. *Ann. Vasc. Surg.* **2014**, *28*, 946–950. [CrossRef] [PubMed]
25. George, R.S.; Milton, R.; Chaudhuri, N.; Kefaloyannis, E.; Papagiannopoulos, K.; Thorax, M. Totally Endoscopic (VATS) First Rib Resection for Thoracic Outlet Syndrome. *Ann. Thorac. Surg.* **2016**, *8*, E1739. [CrossRef] [PubMed]
26. Soukiasian, H.J.; Shouhed, D.; Serna-Gallgos, D.; McKenna, R.; Bairamian, V.J.; McKenna, R.J. A Video-Assisted Thoracoscopic Approach to Transaxillary First Rib Resection. *Innov. Technol. Tech. Cardiothorac. Vasc. Surg.* **2015**, *10*, 21–26. [CrossRef] [PubMed]
27. Gharagozloo, F.; Meyer, M.; Tempesta, B.J.; Margolis, M.; Strother, E.T.; Tummala, S. Robotic en bloc first-rib resection for Paget-Schroetter disease, a form of thoracic outlet syndrome: Technique and initial results. *Innov. Technol. Tech. Cardiothorac. Vasc. Surg.* **2012**, *7*, 39–44. [CrossRef] [PubMed]
28. Meyer, M.; Nguyen, D.; Moslemi, M.; Tempesta, B.; Maas, K.; Poston, R.; Gharagozloo, F. Robotic first rib resection for the treatment of thoracic outlet syndrome: Redefining diagnosis and treatment. *Innov. Technol. Tech. Cardiothorac. Vasc. Surg.* **2014**, *9*, 182–183.
29. de León, R.A.; Chang, D.C.; Hassoun, H.T.; Black, J.H.; Roseborough, G.S.; Perler, B.A.; Rotellini-Coltvet, L.; Call, D. Multiple treatment algorithms for successful outcomes in venous thoracic outlet syndrome. *Surgery* **2009**, *145*, 500–507. [CrossRef] [PubMed]
30. Candia-de las Rosa, R.F.; Perez-Rodriguez, A.; Candia-Garcia, R.; Palacios-Solis, J.M. Endoscopic transaxillary first rib resection for thoracic outlet syndrome: A safe surgical option. *Cir. Cir.* **2010**, *78*, 53–59.
31. Franklin, G.; Fulton-Kehoe, D.; Bradley, C.; Smith-Weller, T. Outcome of surgery for thoracic outlet syndrome in Washington state workers' compensation. *Neurology.* **2000**, *54*, 1252–1257. [CrossRef] [PubMed]
32. Freischlag, J.; Orion, K. Understanding thoracic outlet syndrome. *Scientifica* **2014**. [CrossRef] [PubMed]
33. Chandra, V.; Little, C.; Lee, J.T. Thoracic outlet syndrome in high-performance athletes. *J. Vasc. Surg.* **2014**, *60*, 1012–1018. [CrossRef] [PubMed]
34. Lee, G.W.; Kwon, Y.H.; Jeong, J.H.; Kim, J.W. The efficacy of scalene injection in thoracic outlet syndrome. *J. Korean Neurosurg. Soc.* **2011**, *50*, 36–39. [CrossRef] [PubMed]
35. Finlayson, H.C.; O'Connor, R.J.; Brasher, P.M.A.; Travlos, A. Botulinum toxin injection for management of thoracic outlet syndrome: A double-blind, randomized, controlled trial. *Pain* **2011**, *152*, 2023–2028. [CrossRef] [PubMed]

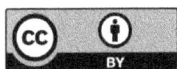

diagnostics

MDPI

Review

Vascular TOS—Creating a Protocol and Sticking to It

Meena Archie * and David Rigberg *

Division of Vascular Surgery, Department of Surgery,
Ronald Reagan Medical Center at the University of California, Los Angeles, CA 90095, USA
* Correspondence: marchie@mednet.ucla.edu (M.A.); drigberg@mednet.ucla.edu (D.R.); Tel.: +1-310-206-6294

Academic Editors: Julie Ann Freischlag and Natalia O. Glebova
Received: 17 March 2017; Accepted: 4 June 2017; Published: 10 June 2017

Abstract: Thoracic Outlet Syndrome (TOS) describes a set of disorders that arise from compression of the neurovascular structures that exit the thorax and enter the upper extremity. This can present as one of three subtypes: neurogenic, venous, or arterial. The objective of this section is to outline our current practice at a single, high-volume institution for venous and arterial TOS. VTOS: Patients who present within two weeks of acute deep vein thrombosis (DVT) are treated with anticoagulation, venography, and thrombolysis. Those who present later are treated with a transaxillary first rib resection, then a two-week post-operative venoplasty. All patients are anticoagulated for 2 weeks after the post-operative venogram. Those with recurrent thrombosis or residual subclavian vein stenosis undergo repeat thrombolysis or venoplasty, respectively. ATOS: In patients with acute limb ischemia, we proceed with thrombolysis or open thrombectomy if there is evidence of prolonged ischemia. We then perform a staged transaxillary first rib resection followed by reconstruction of the subclavian artery. Patients who present with claudication undergo routine arterial duplex and CT angiogram to determine the pathology of the subclavian artery. They then undergo decompression and subclavian artery repair in a similar staged manner.

Keywords: thoracic outlet syndrome (TOS); thoracic outlet syndrome; vascular TOS (VTOS); arterial TOS (ATOS)

---

1. Introduction

Thoracic Outlet Syndrome (TOS) is a general term used to describe various disorders that arise from compression of neurological or vascular structures that exit the thorax to enter the upper extremity. The thoracic outlet is comprised of the narrow aperture created by the first rib, surrounding musculature and the clavicle. Together, these structures surround the subclavian vein, artery and brachial plexus as they travel distally to the arm. These disorders, as a whole, are rare. The three main forms in decreasing prevalence are neurogenic, venous (also known as Paget Schroetter Syndrome) and arterial. Though uncommon, this disorder is one that all vascular surgeons will encounter at some point, and it is imperative to not only be able to diagnose but also manage these patients.

Doctors have long recognized the occurrence of compressive symptoms due to the anatomical constraints at the thoracic outlet. Historical literature illustrates that this association dates back to Galen's study of cervical ribs. In the early 19th century, Sir Astley Cooper studied the thoracic outlet in relation to subclavian artery aneurysms. Gruber, Coote, Mayo, Halsted, Paget, and Schroetter are just a few additional names on the long list of historical anatomists and surgeons who recognized the compression of the thoracic outlet and its effects on the neighboring neurovasculature. In 1956, Peet coined the term TOS, and the initial first rib resection was performed in 1962 by Clagett. The transaxillary approach can be attributed to Roos, who was inspired by the transaxillary sympathectomy.

It is estimated that 5000 patients are affected by TOS per year worldwide and 3000 operations are performed annually for this condition. The anatomy of the thoracic outlet predisposes the body to this syndrome given the numerous vital structures that traverse a relatively small aperture. The thoracic outlet is comprised of the area created by the edge of the first rib inferiorly, the clavicle and subclavius muscle superiorly and anteriorly, and the anterior and middle scalenes laterally and posteriorly. The subclavian vein is first to exit from an anterior perspective, just lateral to the subclavius muscle. The anterior scalene then inserts into the first rib and sits between the subclavian vein and artery. Next come the subclavian artery and brachial plexus. Finally, the middle scalene muscle is typically the final compressive structure in the thoracic outlet [1].

Based on the subtype of TOS, variations of pathology exist. Venous TOS commonly presents with hypertrophied anterior scalene and subclavius muscles, as patients are typically younger and more muscular. Arterial TOS is typically seen in patients with bony prominences or by additional structures such as a cervical rib [2].

There are several less common anomalies that have been discovered, and the most thorough classification system that exists is likely that of Roos. In this system, there are ten anatomical variations that lead to TOS, which include cervical ribs, additional or prominent tendons, and additional accessory muscles such as the scalenus minimus.

2. Diagnosis of Paget-Schroetter Syndrome

Venous TOS, or Paget-Schroetter Syndrome, typically presents as a sudden-onset phenomenon in an otherwise healthy patient. The typical patient is young, athletic, and might even develop symptoms after a rigorous work out leading to the term "effort thrombosis". Examples include weight lifters, swimmers, volleyball players, and baseball players. The right side is affected in 60–80% of patients [3].

Clinical evaluation for the Paget-Schroetter patient begins with history and physical examination. The history is quite consistent—a healthy, young patient with complaints of sudden swelling of the entire upper extremity. Discomfort, heaviness, and cyanosis are not uncommon. Patients are typically between the ages of 14 and 45, and are usually involved in a work or leisure-related activity with repetitive movements overhead. It is important to note that venous TOS may occur in both athletes and non-athletes. Some studies show that males are affected at a rate of 2:1 versus women [3]. On physical examination, the affected arm is edematous and sometimes cyanotic. Patients often have obvious collateral veins across their shoulder, neck, or chest. The most common presentations are visible collateral veins across the shoulder (99%), upper extremity edema (96%), bluish discoloration (94%), and aching pain with exertion (33%) [4,5].

It is important to develop an efficacious pathway in the management of TOS given the rarity of the disease. In the following sections, we will outline an algorithm that we have found useful in effectively treating TOS.

Once the diagnosis is entertained, we perform a venous duplex. Given the location of the thrombosis, it may be difficult for the ultrasonographer to demonstrate a DVT. Overall, however, this test is highly sensitive and specific in the diagnosis of axillo-subclavian DVT, with sensitivity approaching 97% and specificity approaching 96% [6]. A negative study does not rule out vascular TOS (VTOS) despite these high values. It is important to note that upper extremity DVTs place the patient at risk for pulmonary embolism. However, due to the mechanical compression, it is uncommon that Paget-Schroetter patients suffer from clinically significant pulmonary emboli [7]. Following a positive duplex scan, or if the clinical suspicion is high, we initiate anti-coagulation. If there is an unavoidable delay before imaging can be performed, we will start anticoagulation before the diagnostic work up is completed.

Once the upper extremity DVT is diagnosed and anticoagulation is begun, we proceed to definitive imaging; the vast majority of patients undergo catheter-based venography. However, the diagnosis can also be confirmed with CT or MR venography. When possible, we perform the initial diagnostic venogram with the intention of treating.

3. Management of Paget-Schroetter Syndrome

Following the confirmation of the diagnosis with contrast-enhanced imaging, the patient is a candidate for thrombolysis, especially if the diagnosis has been made within 3 weeks. Access is typically achieved by ultrasound guidance of the ipsilateral basilic vein. Our preferred method is to access the basilic vein with a 4F micropuncture needle, then upsize to a short 5F sheath. Thrombolysis is typically achieved by catheter placement (i.e., McNamara infusion catheter, Covidien, Ireland) in the subclavian vein and infusion of a thrombolytic agent, such as tissue plasminogen activator (Alteplase, Genentech, CA, USA). Our preference is to run the tPA at 0.5 mg/kg/h, though this should be titrated both to clot burden on venography and to serial fibrinogen levels. We maintain the fibrinogen level above 200 mg/dL or >50% of the patient's pre-operative level. Heparin is also infused at a rate of 400 units/h through the sheath to maintain patency. Serial partial thromboplastin times are drawn every six hours to avoid supra-therapeutic heparin infusion. Thrombolysis typically lasts for 48 to 72 h with lysis checks every 24 h. Once patency has been achieved, lysis is completed and the sheath is removed from the basilic vein. The patient is then placed on therapeutic anticoagulation.

It is important to note that not all groups proceed with thrombolysis prior to surgical decompression. A recent study demonstrated that preoperative thrombolysis did not provide benefit compared to simple anticoagulation [8]. The retrospective study analyzed 110 patients who suffered from acute subclavian vein thrombosis. Forty-five of these patients underwent thrombolysis and sixty-five were treated with anticoagulation alone. In both groups, 91% were ultimately patent with symptom improvement. Since there was no significant difference between the two groups, the efficacy of thrombolysis was brought into question and further investigation is warranted. However, this study focused on subacute and chronic presentations of VTOS. Clinical acumen must be exercised, as thrombolysis has shown benefit in treatment of acute subclavian vein thrombosis in VTOS patients.

Once patency of the subclavian vein is established, consideration is given to resection of the first rib. It is now widely accepted that anticoagulation alone is not sufficient for the treatment of venous TOS [9,10]. Historically, successful thrombolysis was followed by three months of therapeutic anticoagulation, after which a trans-axillary first rib resection and scalenectomy were performed as originally described by Kunkel and Machleder [7]. This three-month period from the time of thrombolysis to the first rib resection may increase the risk of re-thrombosis [1,10,11]. The current standard of care is to minimize this waiting period; many even advocate immediate decompression during the same hospitalization [1,10]. It is our current practice to discuss the timing with the patient. We frequently perform rib resection during the initial hospitalization, but can certainly delay operation if the patient has a need to delay it.

Following first rib resection, it is common to have residual stenosis of the subclavian vein due to fibrous strictures or post-thrombotic changes. Reviews of post-operative venograms indicate that approximately 30–45% of patients have such residual lesions [11]. Our preference is to image patients with catheter-based venography and intra-vascular ultrasound (IVUS) two weeks following surgical decompression. In our experience, IVUS provides three-dimensional imaging of the degree of stenosis, which aids in decision-making. We continue anti-coagulation from the postoperative period until we perform these studies. If we find residual venous disease, we perform a venoplasty at the time. Our experience shows that the majority of lysed veins remain patent on post-operative venography, though this has not been studied. If no lesions are found at the 2-week postoperative venogram, we discontinue anticoagulation. If there is residual stenosis, we continue anticoagulation for 2–4 weeks. At this point, we repeat imaging. Only after we have demonstrated a healthy appearing vein 2–4 weeks following an intervention do we stop the anticoagulation. If we are unable to achieve this result after repeated attempts, we will discuss with the patient with the recommendation to continue anticoagulation for up to 12 months to allow for possible improvement in the vein, including the possibility of late recanalization [3].

There is also a sub-group of patients who will thrombose their axillo-subclavian vein between the time of first rib resection and follow up venography. It is essential to consider incomplete decompression as the etiology. Our approach to these patients is to repeat lysis as necessary after the rib has been removed. Venography with IVUS during the lysis completion procedure should reveal a decompressed thoracic outlet. If this is not the case, the patient should be considered for reoperation [12]. At this point, the patients follow the algorithm for post rib resection vein management. (Algorithm A1). Finally, there is a group of patients who experience repeat thrombosis of their axillo-subclavian vein in the interval from the original lysis to rib resection. This occurs in about 34 percent of patients, though the number is thought to have decreased with the increased utilization of lysis and rib resection at the same hospitalization [13,14]. We proceed with rib resection in these patients, and then perform repeated lysis as necessary. Again, the patients are then on our algorithm for the post-rib excision vein management as above.

Although post- first rib resection subclavian vein stenting remains the subject of ongoing review, we avoid the use of stents in this location. It is important to note that this is in reference to post-surgical stenting as opposed to subclavian vein stenting in the non-decompressed thoracic outlet, which has been widely rejected [4,5].

4. Management of Chronic Subclavian Vein Thrombosis in Paget-Schroetter Syndrome

Although there is no definitive length of time for chronic versus acute subclavian vein thrombosis, many authors define acute as less than two weeks and chronic as greater than two weeks [15]. In our experience, surgical decompression takes precedence in the management of patients with symptoms that have been present greater than 3 weeks. We initiate therapeutic anticoagulation in the outpatient setting. Trans-axillary first rib resection is then performed, usually within 2–4 weeks of starting anticoagulation. Two weeks post-operatively, a venogram is performed along with any required intervention including mechanical, on-table, or extended thrombolysis [16,17]. Mechanical thrombolysis yields mixed results, but may be beneficial about 50% of the time [8]. There is not much data regarding on-table lysis; however, we opt to use this technique in patients with residual thrombosis after decompression if the thrombus is relatively small in appearance and the residual stenosis is minimal. If a more significant thrombus burden is seen, extended lysis is performed as described above. It is also accepted that the subclavian vein may recanalize after decompression alone, even if it remains occluded following surgical decompression [17]. This is further reason for decompressing patients who have had a more long-standing occlusion of the axillo-subclavian vein. Again, our protocol is to continue anti-coagulation until a patent, healthy-appearing vein is demonstrated on follow up imaging—typically two weeks after the last intervention. If this cannot be attained, we continue anticoagulation for several months to encourage spontaneous clot resolution.

5. Contralateral Asymptomatic Lesions

A small subgroup of patients will present with unilateral symptoms despite significant compression of the contralateral side on imaging. We favor treating a very small minority of these patients with decompression prophylactically, though we recognize this is controversial and is not supported by the literature. Transaxillary first rib resection is our preferred method in these patients as well.

6. Venous Reconstruction and Other Surgical Techniques

A small subgroup of Paget-Schroetter patients will require further surgery after venoplasty, thrombolysis, and conventional surgical decompression fail to correct their symptoms. It is important to stress that these procedures should only be considered in patients with persistent and disabling symptoms from an occluded axillo-subclavian vein. The final end point should be symptom status, not necessarily radiologic patency of the subclavian vein. In the rare cases where open venous reconstruction is needed, we have used an infraclavicular approach with placement of an interposition graft. It is essential to ensure that the venous inflow from the brachial vein is adequate to maintain patency of the repair. The best choice of graft is native vein, such as the saphenous. The patient is typically maintained on 3–6 months of anticoagulation afterwards [18].

7. VTOS Case Presentation

An otherwise healthy 36 year-old female athlete presented to an outside hospital with an acutely swollen right arm. Acute right axillosubclavian vein thrombosis was diagnosed by a combination of duplex ultrasound imaging and venography. She underwent thrombolysis at that hospital, then presented to us for further management. She had been anticoagulated with Rivaroxaban.

She underwent venography of the right arm venous system which revealed a 70–80% stenosis of the right subclavian vein in neutral position (Figures 1 and 2). The vein was completely occluded in stress position. This was confirmed with intra-vascular ultrasound (IVUS). On IVUS measurements, the neutral position yielded a 74.4% stenosis while the stress position yielded 100% total occlusion (Figures 3 and 4). It was noted that the contralateral vein appeared compressed in the costochondral space as well, though she was asymptomatic.

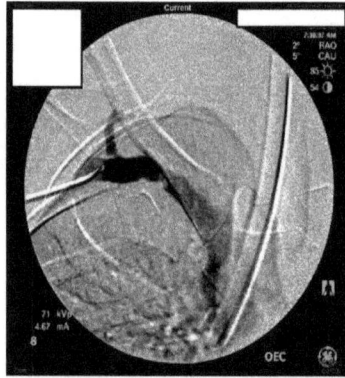

Figure 1. Venogram of a Paget-Schroetter patient in the stress position demonstrating significant stenosis of the right subclavian vein.

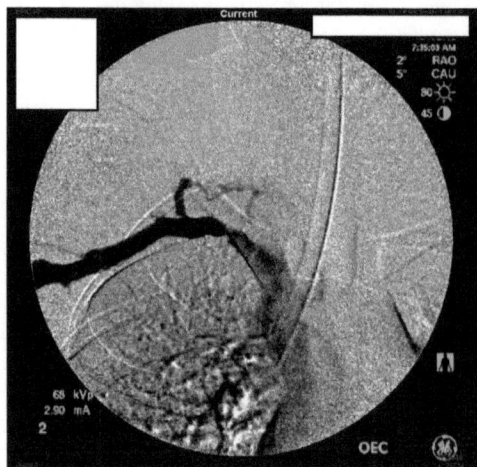

Figure 2. Venogram demonstrating a right subclavian vein that is nearly occluded while in stress position.

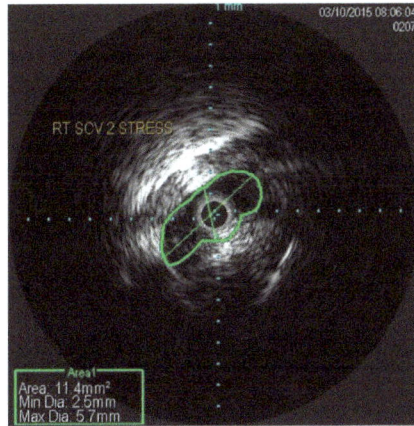

Figure 3. Nearly occluded right subclavian vein in stress position as demonstrated by IVUS.

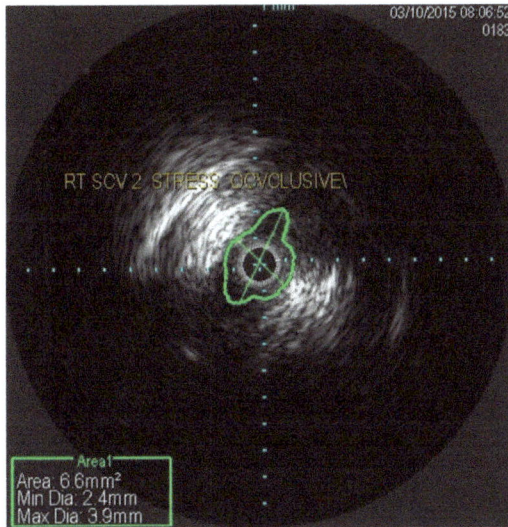

Figure 4. Occlusion of the right subclavian vein in stress position as demonstrated by IVUS.

She underwent trans-axillary first rib resection. She recovered quickly and was discharged two days post-operatively. She resumed Rivaroxaban on post-operative day 5. She was brought back for a post-operative venogram with IVUS two weeks post-operatively. This revealed a high grade stenosis of the subclavian vein at the thoracic outlet. The lesion was treated with a 12 mm diameter balloon, which was effective.

A left-sided venogram was performed simultaneously, which revealed high-grade stenosis of the subclavian vein at the thoracic outlet. She was brought back two months afterwards for a trans-axillary first rib resection given the significant compression on venography and IVUS. It is important to note that treatment of the contralateral side is not widely accepted. However, we opted to proceed after a thorough discussion with the patient regarding her alternatives. She was kept on anticoagulation one month post-operatively, then discontinued. She was followed for up to one year post-operatively with no recurrence of symptoms and full resolution of normal activity.

8. Diagnosis of Arterial Thoracic Outlet Syndrome

Arterial thoracic outlet syndrome (ATOS) is a rare phenomenon typically seen in young, healthy individuals. It is frequently a result of a bony anomaly leading to subclavian artery compression and repetitive trauma. This results in arterial changes including aneurysmal dilatation, stenosis, or ulceration. The anatomical changes that typically cause ATOS include the cervical rib, anomaly of the first rib, or bony spurs that result from previous bone fractures [19,20]. The incidence of ATOS in TOS patients is approximately 6% [5].

Clinical presentation of ATOS is similar to arterial sufficiency in any extremity. The spectrum of symptoms ranges from effort fatigue to subacute or acute limb ischemia, which occur in approximately 50% of patients [21]. Rarely, posterior stroke symptoms may occur (approximately 5% of patients). If significant aneurysmal degeneration has occurred, a pulsatile mass in the shoulder or upper chest may be described (15% of patients) [21]. History typically includes repetitive overhead activity, and subtle physical exam findings may include splinter hemorrhages distally.

Our experience indicates that a subclavian artery duplex is a valuable initial study once the diagnosis of ATOS is suspected. Duplex ultrasonography allows for the visualization of the artery and provides vital information including the size of the artery, flow characteristics, presence or absence of thrombosis, and distal perfusion. We then obtain a CTA of the affected extremity to assist in operative planning; however, this study is sometimes omitted if the duplex has provided this information. Our gold standard for diagnosis is catheter-based angiography, although modern MR and CT angiography allows for avoidance of catheter-based procedures unless there is also an intention to treat. Essential findings include aneurysmal or ulcerative degeneration, size of lesion, mural thrombus, and distal emboli [5,17].

9. Management of Arterial Thoracic Outlet Syndrome

Management of ATOS is dictated by the presentation. Acute arm ischemia in these patients is treated first. If the ischemia is not limb-threatening, thrombolysis is performed, especially if there is evidence of thrombosis in the digital arteries as these are difficult to treat surgically. Thrombolysis follows the same principles outlined above. Access is achieved by femoral or radial approach depending on arch anatomy. Our preferred method is to with a 4F micropuncture needle, then upsize to a short 5F sheath. A catheter is placed within the target vessel, and Alteplase (Genentech) is infused at a rate of 0.5 mg/kg/h while heparin runs through the access sheath at 400 units/hr. Serial PTTs and fibrinogen levels are followed. Lysis checks are performed under angiography every 24 h while strict neurovascular checks are performed every two hours in the intensive care unit.

If the patient presents with acute limb-threatening ischemia, these patients are emergently taken to the operating room for exploration and open thrombectomy. The operative approach depends on the site of arterial occlusion. This can be determined by a combination of physical examination and noninvasive/radiographic findings. Emboli frequently lodge at branch points, and it is common to have a cutoff in the brachial artery. If imaging suggests a limited embolus, a simple cut-down and embolectomy at the brachial artery can be performed. Retrograde approaches to clot removal can also be performed from a brachial approach. Using careful technique, clot can also be removed from the radial and ulnar arteries via a brachial approach. On-table angiography is then performed; if residual thrombus is seen, simultaneous thrombolysis can be performed. There are occasions where consideration must be given to upper extremity fasciotomies, so the limb should be carefully evaluated following revascularization.

Once the upper extremity is revascularized, we continue the patient on therapeutic anticoagulation while a definitive plan is made for decompression and arterial reconstruction. Bony anomalies are the typical etiology in ATOS—more so than the venous or neurogenic subtypes. For these issues, a first rib resection or resection of the bony prominence is essential. The presence of a cervical rib can be as high as 75% of patients. In these patients, we prefer to resect both the first and cervical ribs by supraclavicular approach. In approximately 12% of patients, a first rib abnormality alone is the issue;

in these patients, we opt for a transaxillary first rib resection [21]. Repairing the subclavian artery is performed at a later stage by supraclavicular approach. Other bony prominences such as a healed clavicular fracture occur in less than 10% of patients. In these circumstances, we perform a first rib resection in addition to resection of the bony prominence [21].

10. Approach to Subclavian Artery Repair in ATOS

The supraclavicular approach provides excellent exposure to all anatomic structures associated with the thoracic outlet. It is useful in repairing the subclavian artery in ATOS patients and provides the possibility of simultaneous decompression, though we prefer a staged approach in order to ensure a complete first rib resection.

With the patient in supine position and a transverse roll placed beneath the shoulders, the sternal notch, clavicle, and sternocleidomastoid muscle are identified. A transverse incision is made 1 cm superior to the clavicle just lateral to the sternocleidomastoid. Dissection through the subcutaneous tissue and platysma is performed. The external jugular will be encountered and should be ligated. The sternocleidomastoid is then divided. This should be performed carefully, as the carotid sheath lies directly beneath. This dissection should be carried out carefully on the left side to avoid injuring the thoracic duct as well, which drains at the confluence of the internal jugular and subclavian veins.

The scalene fat pad is then dissected along the medial border and reflected laterally to expose the anterior scalene muscle. The phrenic nerve is carefully identified, and the scalene muscle transected. Once transected, the subclavian artery will be easily visualized [22]. Once exposed, the artery may be repaired with a biologic interposition graft, direct primary repair, or ligation and distal bypass. These options have similar patency rates as well as patient functionality outcomes [21].

In terms of endovascular approaches, there is a paucity for data for the use of covered stents in the subclavian artery in ATOS. Historically, subclavian artery stents have a low 1-year patency rate, as low as 60% when used for aneurysm repair [23]. We have occasionally utilized this technique for ATOS patients. In one case, a young, athletic patient with a subclavian artery aneurysm from ATOS was treated with a covered stent (Viabahn, Gore, Flagstaff, AZ, USA), which remained patent for 9 years while on aspirin. The stent occluded and he presented with acute arm ischemia, which was successfully treated with thrombolysis. The secondary patency period is yet to be determined. In a different case, a young woman was also treated with an endograft (Viabahn), which remained patent for two years. She then returned with recurrent claudication and significant in-stent restenosis requiring angioplasty with a drug-eluting balloon. Though we have not investigated this data closely, it is likely that long-term patency of this technique may be inferior to traditional reconstruction.

11. Contralateral Asymptomatic Lesions

As in VTOS patients, a subgroup present with unilateral symptoms while having marked compression of the contralateral side on imaging. We favor treating these patients with decompression prophylactically, though we realize this is disputed. Transaxillary first rib resection is our preferred method in these patients as well.

12. ATOS Case Presentation

A 27 year-old female who had suffered a left clavicular fracture that was repaired previously presented with left upper extremity numbness and pain for one week. The symptoms occurred spontaneously and were intermittent throughout the week. She experienced no relief with analgesics. She presented to our Emergency Department. Brachial, ulnar and radial pulses were non-palpable. An arterial duplex revealed an occlusive thrombus of the brachial artery at the mid-humerus that appeared to be associated with the patient's previous clavicular repair (Figure 5). A CT angiogram subsequently revealed a subclavian artery aneurysm adjacent to one of the screws from her prior clavicle repair (Figure 6).

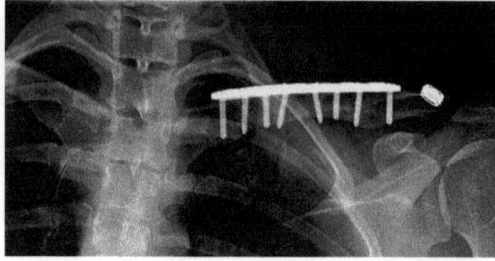

Figure 5. Arterial thoracic outlet syndrome (ATOS) patient with metal plate and screws after a prior clavicular fracture—the screws are abutting the thoracic outlet.

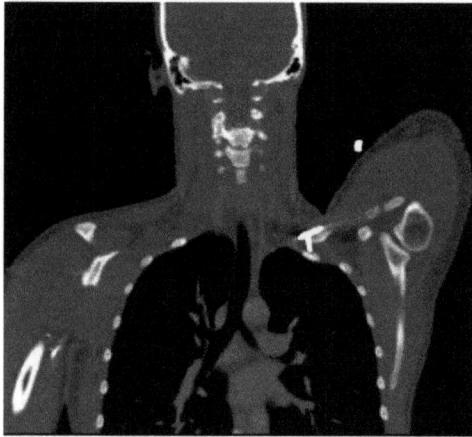

Figure 6. CT angiogram demonstrating a screw abutting the thoracic outlet in an ATOS patient with a subclavian artery aneurysm.

A heparin drip was then initiated, and she was taken to the catheterization lab for thrombolysis. This was carried out with Alteplase for 48 h as the patient had strong collaterals and was not in limb-threat (Figures 7–11). However, her radial artery remained occluded. She was then taken to the operating room for thromboembolectomy of the left brachial and radial arteries (Figure 12). She was continued on anticoagulation post-operatively and was discharged.

Two months later, she was brought in for a trans-axillary left first rib resection and a placement of a 7 mm by 5 cm Viabahn endograft to exclude the subclavian aneurysm. Anticoagulation was withheld 3 days prior to the operation. Orthopedic Surgery was consulted to remove the adjacent screws simultaneously. She was discharged on Aspirin and Plavix two days post-operatively.

She was followed every six weeks for 18 weeks, then every 3 months the first year. She received arterial duplex ultrasounds at the 3-month, 6-month, and 12-month intervals for the first year. These revealed mild in-stent restenosis, which was stable.

She presented nearly two years later with recurrent left arm claudication. An angiogram revealed a significant in-stent restenosis that was significantly flow-limiting. This was treated with a 6 mm × 4 cm paclitaxel-coated balloon. Her symptoms improved, and she has been followed up to over 18 months after the secondary intervention without symptoms. A discussion was held as to whether treatment of the contralateral side was warranted. We did not proceed with treatment, as she was asymptomatic and compression of the right side was not demonstrated to the same degree as the left. As mentioned earlier, treatment of contralateral limbs is not widely accepted and should only be done after a thorough discussion with the patient regarding the efficacy of further intervention.

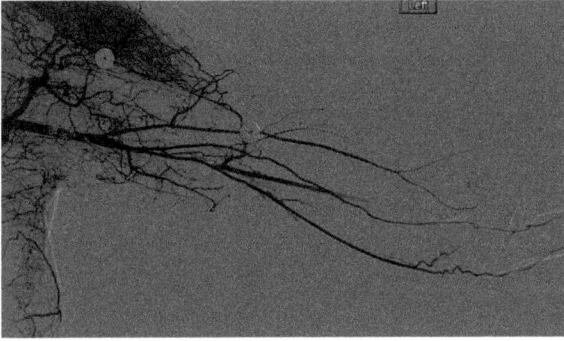

Figure 7. Left subclavian arteriography demonstrating a thrombosed brachial artery at the mid-humeral level and extensive collateralization proximally.

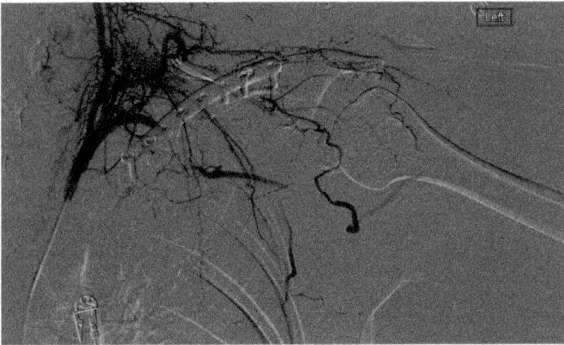

Figure 8. Left subclavian arteriography in an ATOS patient in stress position demonstrating a totally occluded subclavian artery.

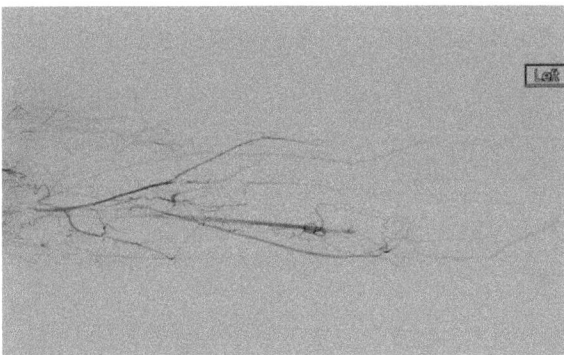

Figure 9. Distal left arm angiography in an ATOS patient demonstrating an occluded radial artery at the origin and ulnar artery at the mid-forearm.

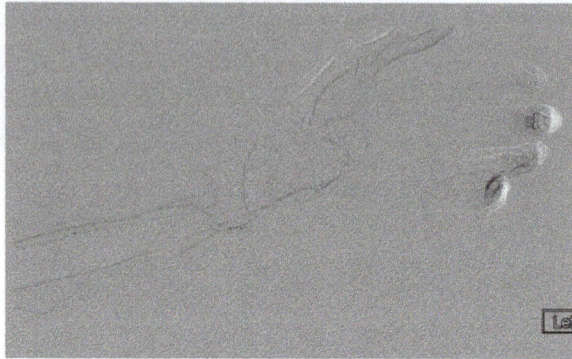

Figure 10. Angiography of the radial and ulnar arteries as well as the palmar arch and digital branches in an ATOS patient with a brachial thrombus.

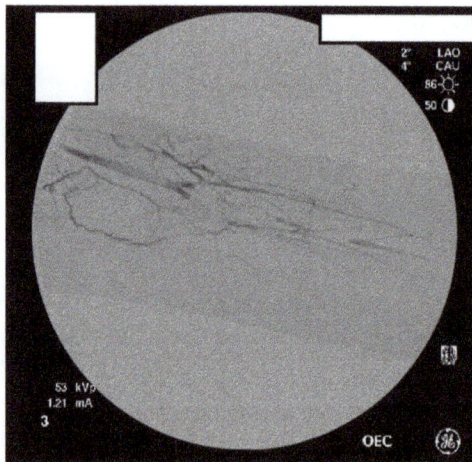

Figure 11. Distal brachial artery thrombosis in an ATOS patient.

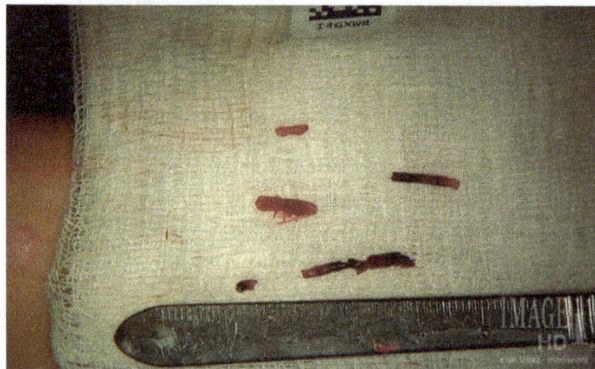

Figure 12. Excised thrombus from the brachial and radial arteries of an ATOS patient with a subclavian artery aneurysm.

13. Conclusions

Vascular thoracic outlet syndrome is a rare disorder. The principles of managing venous TOS revolve around decompression and keeping the subclavian vein patent, if possible. These include early diagnosis, swift thrombolysis, and transaxillary decompression. More importantly, it is essential to commit to an efficacious algorithm such as the one outlined in this paper. Work up typically begins with duplex ultrasound and is followed by venography and thrombolysis or a first rib resection depending on the findings. This is followed by a two-week post-operative venogram and anticoagulation for one month. Patients with persistent symptoms are treated with repeated efforts of thrombolysis (Figure A1).

Managing arterial TOS depends on the presentation of the patient. The degree of ischemia may dictate a rapid, open approach to the arterial compromise, although many patients can safely undergo thrombolysis. Lytic therapy is much more likely to allow for complete resolution of the distal thrombus that can occur in these patients. As with venous TOS, definitive therapy requires decompression of the thoracic outlet and ultimately, repair of the injured vessel (Figure A2).

Conflicts of Interest: The authors declare no conflict of interest.

Appendix A

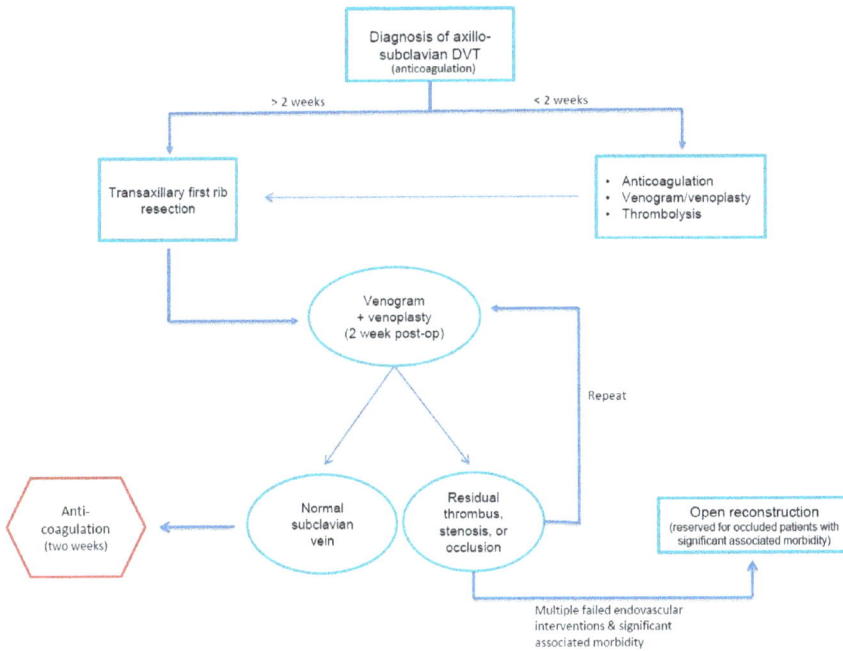

Figure A1. VTOS.

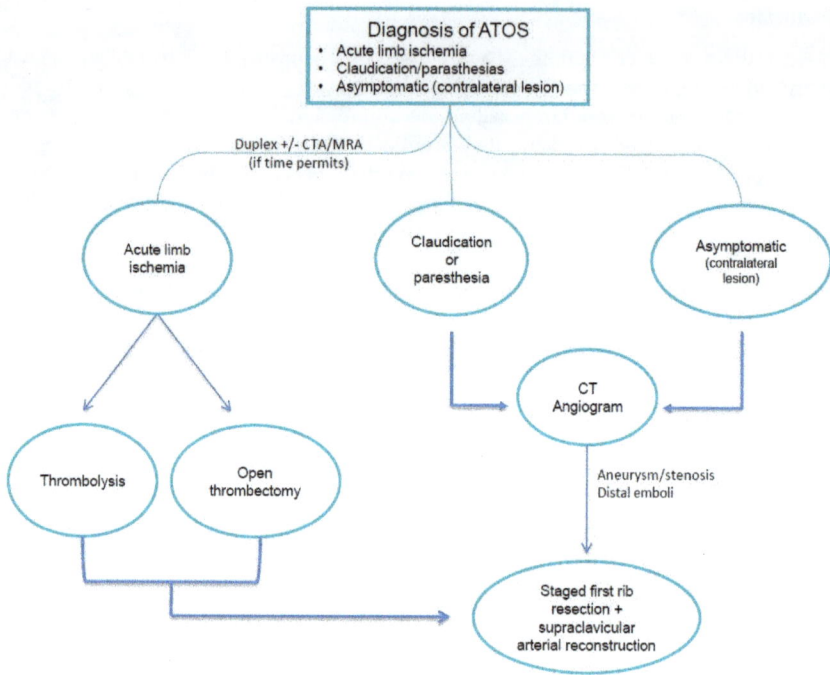

Figure A2. ATOS.

References

1. Urschel, H.C.; Razzuk, M.A. Paget-Schroetter syndrome: What is the best management? *Ann. Thorac. Surg.* **2000**, *69*, 1663–1669. [CrossRef]
2. Hussain, M.A.; Al-Omran, M. Vascular Thoracic Outlet Syndrome. *Semin. Thorac. Surg.* **2016**, *28*, 151–157. [CrossRef] [PubMed]
3. Lindblad, B.; Bergqvist, D. Deep vein thrombosis of the axillary-subclavian veins: Epidemiologic data, effects of different types of treatment and late sequelae. *Eur. J. Vasc. Surg.* **1988**, *2*, 561–567. [CrossRef]
4. Urschel, J.C., Jr.; Patel, A.N. Paget-Schroetter syndrome therapy: Failure of intravenous stents. *Ann. Thorac. Surg.* **2003**, *75*, 1693–1696. [CrossRef]
5. Urschel, H.C.; Kourlis, H. Thoracic outlet syndrome: A 50-year experience at Baylor University Medical Center. *Proceedings* **2007**, *20*, 125–135.
6. Di Nisio, M.; Van Sluis, G.L.; Bossuyt, P.M.; Büller, H.R.; Porreca, E.; Rutjes, A.W. Accuracy of diagnostic tests for clinically suspected upper extremity deep vein thrombosis: A systematic review. *J. Thromb. Haemost.* **2010**, *8*, 684–692. [CrossRef] [PubMed]
7. Hobeika, C.; Lababede, O. Paget-Schroetter syndrome: An uncommon cause of pulmonary embolic disease. *J. Thorac. Imaging* **2010**, *25*, 1–3. [CrossRef] [PubMed]
8. Guzzo, J.L.; Freischlag, J.A. Preoperative thrombolysis and venoplasty affords no benefit in patency following first rib resection and scalenectomy for subacute and chronic subclavian vein thrombosis. *J. Vasc. Surg.* **2010**, *52*, 658–662. [CrossRef] [PubMed]
9. Lee, J.T.; Karwowski, J.K.; Harris, E.J.; Haukoos, J.S.; Olcott, C., IV. Long-term thrombotic recurrence after nonoperative management of Paget-Schroetter syndrome. *J. Vasc. Surg.* **2006**, *43*, 1236–1243. [CrossRef] [PubMed]
10. Molina, J.E.; Hunter, D.W.; Dietz, C.A. Paget-Schroetter syndrome treated with thrombolytics and immediate surgery. *J. Vasc. Surg.* **2007**, *45*, 328–334. [CrossRef] [PubMed]

Diagnostics **2017**, *7*, 34

11. Angle, N.; Gelabert, H.A.; Farooq, M.M.; Ahn, S.S.; Caswell, D.R.; Freischlag, J.A.; Machleder, H.I. Safety and efficacy of early surgical decompression of thoracic outlet for Paget-Schroetter syndrome. *Ann. Vasc. Surg.* **2001**, *15*, 37–42. [CrossRef] [PubMed]

12. Molina, J.E. Reoperations after failed transaxillary first rib resection to treat Paget-Schroetter syndrome patients. *Ann. Thorac. Surg.* **2011**, *91*, 1717–1722. [CrossRef] [PubMed]

13. Machleder, H.I. Evaluation of a new treatment strategy for Paget-Schroetter syndrome: Spontaneous thrombosis of the axillary–subclavian vein. *J. Vasc. Surg.* **1993**, *17*, 305–315. [CrossRef]

14. Lee, M.C.; Belkin, M. Early operative intervention after thrombolytic therapy for primary subclavian vein thrombosis: An effective treatment approach. *J. Vasc. Surg.* **1998**, *27*, 1101–1108. [CrossRef]

15. Illig, K.A.; Doyle, A.J. A comprehensive review of Paget-Schroetter syndrome. *J. Vasc. Surg.* **2010**, *51*, 1538–1547. [CrossRef] [PubMed]

16. Caparrelli, D.J.; Freischlag, J.A. A unified approach to axillosubclavian venous thrombosis in a single hospital admission. *Semin. Vasc. Surg.* **2005**, *18*, 153–157. [CrossRef] [PubMed]

17. De Leon, R.A.; Chang, D.C.; Busse, C.; Call, D.; Freischlag, J.A. First rib resection and scalenectomy for chronically occluded subclavian veins: What does it really do? *Ann. Vasc. Surg.* **2008**, *22*, 395–401. [CrossRef] [PubMed]

18. Sanders, R.J.; Haug, C. Subclavian vein obstruction and thoracic outlet syndrome: A review of etiology and management. *Ann. Vasc. Surg.* **1990**, *4*, 397–410. [CrossRef] [PubMed]

19. Durham, J.R.; Yao, J.S.; Pearce, W.H.; McCarthy, W.J., III; Nuber, G.M. Arterial injuries in the thoracic outlet syndrome. *J. Vasc. Surg.* **1995**, *21*, 57–69. [CrossRef]

20. Criado, E.; Greenfield, L. The spectrum of arterial compression at the thoracic outlet. *J. Vasc. Surg.* **2010**, *52*, 406–411. [CrossRef] [PubMed]

21. Vemuri, C.; McLaughlin, L.N.; Abuirqeba, A.A.; Thompson, R.W. Clinical presentation and management of arterial thoracic outlet syndrome. *J. Vasc. Surg.* **2017**, *65*, 1429–1439. [CrossRef] [PubMed]

22. Singh, M.J.; Fanciullo, D.J. Chapter 85: Surgical Techniques: Approach to the Axillosubclavian Artery. In *Thoracic Outlet Syndrome*; Springer-Verlag: London, UK, 2013; pp. 597–600.

23. Rigberg, D.; Freischlag, J.A. Thoracic Outlet Syndrome. In *Comprehensive Vascular and Endovascular Surgery*; Elsevier: Philadelphia, PA, USA, 2004; pp. 318–334.

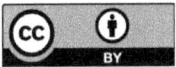

diagnostics

MDPI

Article

Creating a Registry for Patients with Thoracic Outlet Syndrome

Misty D. Humphries

Division of Vascular and Endovascular Surgery, University of California Davis Health, 4860 Y Street, Suite 3400, Sacramento, CA 95817, USA; mdhumphries@ucdavis.edu

Academic Editor: Andreas Kjaer
Received: 3 March 2017; Accepted: 24 May 2017; Published: 17 June 2017

Abstract: The creation of any patient database requires substantial planning. In the case of thoracic outlet syndrome, which is a rare disease, the Society for Vascular Surgery has defined reporting standards to serve as an outline for the creation of a patient registry. Prior to undertaking this task, it is critical that designers understand the basics of registry planning and a priori establish plans for data collection and analysis.

Keywords: Thoracic Outlet Syndrome (TOS); nTOS; aTOS; vTOS; Paget-Schroetter syndrome

---

1. Introduction

A registry is defined as a place where data, records, or laboratory samples are kept and made available for research [1]. Registries have become powerful tools to observe the course of disease, understand variation in treatment and outcomes, describe patterns of care, and examine factors that influence prognosis and quality of life. Registries are particularly useful in the case of rare diseases where the ability to conduct clinical trials is hindered by the rarity of the condition and the aggregation of treatment to specialty centers. Thoracic Outlet Syndrome (TOS) is an example of a rare disease where diagnosis can be extremely challenging, especially in the case of neurogenic TOS. Nuances of treatment and post-operative care are critical to successful outcomes, and there are clear patient and disease characteristics that influence prognosis in TOS. The establishment of a TOS registry allows for aggregation of data, not just at one institution, but across centers, with the goal of comparing treatment and guiding management. Registries have allowed for the development of outcomes standards in rare disease and establish what providers in real-world practice can achieve. The Agency for Healthcare Research and Quality has produced a summary which can provide guidance and answer questions when attempting to create a registry [2].

2. Registry Planning

The creation of a registry begins with defining the purpose of the registry. There are five main purposes for registries: (1) describing the natural history of disease; (2) determining clinical and/or cost-effectiveness; (3) assessing safety or harm; (4) measuring or improving quality of care; (5) public health surveillance and disease control. Multiple studies have demonstrated disparities between results in clinical trials and results in clinical practice [3,4]. Efficacy of treatment for well-defined patient populations in trials may not be generalizable to other populations or subgroups. Improvement in comparative effectiveness methodologies in observational research has increased interest in the investment in registries across many stakeholders. Both the Institute of Medicine (IOM) and the Federal Coordinating Council for Comparative Effectiveness Research have identified patient registries as a core component of comparative effectiveness data infrastructure [5,6]. Registries are also expected to play an important role in the Patient Centered Outcomes Research Institute (PCORI) for their ability to provide information in the "real-world" setting and measure quality of care. Quality-based registries are increasingly able to assess differences between providers and patient populations based on performance measures and identify disparities, demonstrate opportunities for improvement, and provide transparency through public reporting. Most registries are developed with more than one purpose in mind. Additionally, registries designed with an initial purpose may be modified over time to accommodate additional purposes of research, practice, or policy environment changes.

The second step in planning a registry is identifying stakeholders. Stakeholders can play an integral part in design and function of a registry. They are invaluable at ensuring the registry is meeting its key objectives over time. This is particularly important for registries that collect data over many years. Stakeholders include patients, clinicians, providers, product manufacturers, and payers. In rare disease registries, such as TOS, stakeholders may also include advocacy groups, public health agencies, and scientists. Stakeholders are typically classified as primary—those that create and fund the registry—or secondary—those that would benefit from knowledge of the data or would be impacted by the results. Different stakeholders will perceive and benefit from the registry in different ways. For physicians, the registry can provide insight into management of a disease in accordance with evidence-based guidelines [7]. For patients and patient advocacy groups, a registry can increase understanding of the natural history of a disease, contribute to the development of treatment guidelines, or facilitate research on treatment [7,8]. When multiple stakeholders are involved, clear policies should be in place regarding governance, data access, and the publication of data from registries. It is also important that communication with stakeholders is consistent to maintain their interest in success of the registry.

A key element in determining the feasibility of a new registry is funding, which is especially true for national registries. Local registries, where the scope is more limited, may be set up with less expense. Specific factors that determine the feasibility of a registry include the number of sites, number of patients, the scope of data to be collected, and the methods used to collect data. Acquisition of data from the electronic health record through computerized means is highly feasible, but manual extraction of data imbedded in free text fields requires a team of people, which may preclude the collection of large amounts of data. Creating electronic portals into which participants can easily enter their own data at the initial visit and at home for follow-up can improve collection, especially in cases where participants may see multiple clinicians in many different fields. In the case of TOS, patients may see a physical therapist, a pain management specialist, and a surgical specialist. Collection of data from each visit can be facilitated by allowing the registry participant to enter data at home through regular emailed updates. This also improves the likelihood that participants will answer honestly and not be swayed by a provider.

3. Scope

The scope of a registry is viewed in terms of the size, setting, duration, geography, and financing. The purpose and objectives of the registry frame the scope, although other factors, such as research interests and disease specific guidelines, will also shape it. The scope of a registry is also affected by the degree of uncertainty acceptable to primary stakeholders. The amount of uncertainty is determined by weighing the quantity, quality, and detail of the data collected against its considered importance and value. Here, we will focus on two key concepts in scope: the core data set and patient outcomes.

Each data element included in the core data set should address the central questions for which the registry was designed. These should be balanced with noncore variables, such as more descriptive or exploratory ones. Balance is required in the use of core and noncore variables and reduces attempts to accomplish too many goals. When there are excessive noncore data elements, collecting data becomes a significant burden. This ultimately outweighs the usefulness to clinical sites and prevents them from participating. Even when core variables are limited and appear relatively easy to collate, the reliability of some variables can be suspect. The Society for Vascular Surgery has put forth a formal reporting standards document for patients with TOS. This document provides examples of data collection variables and specifics into which variables should be considered core and noncore [9]. Within a TOS registry, for example, the exact use of medications and the variable nature of medication reporting can call into question the reliability of whether patients are using narcotics or illegal substances to control their pain. Finally, consideration of what data are readily available may determine what will remain part of the core data. Data that are consistent with general practice are typically much easier to collect that data that exceed usual practice. This is especially true for quality-of-life data. For patients with TOS, there are multiple data forms that can be used to assess quality of life. Not all institutions can collect data from the Quick-Dash, the SF-12, and a brief pain inventory. Although collection of data from each survey yields more information about the patients' functionality and life, for many practices, quality-of-life data are not an essential element collected in a routine history or physical. In creating our own database, we could have labeled quality-of-life data as a noncore data element. This would allow more institutions to participate, but may limit conclusions that can be made regarding treatment. For this reason, we focus on collecting these patient centered outcomes in order to better refine treatment. Furthermore, because there is not a TOS-specific quality-of-life form, many institutions may use their own forms or select one form over another. In addition to establishment of core and noncore elements, patient outcomes in the order of greatest importance should be identified early in the concept phase of the registry. Defining which outcomes will be primary and secondary forces prioritization within the design of the registry.

4. Data Collection

Data collection is a fluid process that should be pilot tested, adjusted, and retested several times prior to the full implementation of a clinical registry. This process, although onerous, is imperative to the long-term success of the registry. In the case of our registry, testing took 16 months to ensure the ease of use. An initial case report form should be developed. This is a formatted list of data elements that can be presented in paper or electronic form and is the data structure of a clinical registry. The case report form is developed as the purpose and scope are delineated with principles regarding the core and noncore elements, and then it is modified numerous times as the registry is pilot tested. Once the case report form has been conceived, a data dictionary of definitions and parameters should be developed. The data dictionary should describe each data element and provide information about how the data should be interpreted. This is especially important for data which are to be extracted from a chart by research personnel who may not be as knowledgeable about the clinical condition.

The most successful registries utilize a collection system that can be integrated into day-to-day clinical practice. The case report should be broken down by the type of clinical visit; initial evaluation, surgical treatment, non-surgical treatment, and follow-up. Specific data elements tailored for each type of visit, as well as patient reported outcomes, are collected by translating the case report form into a two-part document for the clinician and the patient to complete. Although paper forms may be used, electronic versions of data entry can simplify collection for patients, especially if there are multiple forms. In the case of the Vascular Quality Initiative database, the vast amount of data requires specialized personnel to extract data. In our own TOS database, data are extracted from the electronic medical record through a specific TOS clinical template. The creation of a mobile tablet-based case report form can be used in the waiting room after patients have checked in for their visit. In cases where there are multiple data forms or surveys, the presence of a research assistant may be required to help guide the participant through the data collection process. To simplify data collection by the clinician, the case report form should be converted into an electronic health record clinical documentation template. This allows for easy incorporation into practice and extraction by registry personnel. The paper-based form can be given to the clinician for use in guiding the visit, and then translated into the clinic visit note. This too ensures ease of extracting data for research personnel.

5. Data Analysis

Not all registries are developed with a testable hypothesis in mind, and this is perfectly reasonable. Studies that emerge from registries may initially present descriptive work that has largely been unknown, such as clinical progression. In registries where the aim is to study the association between a specific exposure and outcome, prespecification of the study methodology and the establishment of a prior hypothesis may affect the acceptance of results derived from the registry. On the other hand, a study may evolve out of an unexpected observation in the database during analysis for other purposes, or may evolve from a concerted effort of the registry participants to answer a specific question. Regardless, transparency in methods is essential in order to allow the reader to understand whether the analysis evolved from multiple iterations of exploratory analysis or whether it was a hypothesis developed independently of the registry.

During any analysis of registry data, the first step is to assess the data quality. Missing data can represent a challenge for any registry-based analysis. Missing data can include situations where one question in a group of variables is not answered, such as a patient-reported survey. In this type of case, a decision must be made: should the entire patient record be removed? Or should parts of the data be analyzed as complete while other parts as missing? Removing the record completely reduces the information yield from the study, while analyzing partial records could seriously bias the results. One way to determine whether or not data are missing at random is to compare the distribution of observation variables for patients with specific missing data to the distribution of patients for whom that data are present. Though it may still be difficult to explain why the data are missing, this is an accepted analytical method for managing missing data.

While there are numerous methods of analyzing observational data, the decision to perform a descriptive or comparative analysis is the first step. Statistical methods used for descriptive purposes include summarization of continuous and categorical data, reporting incidence and prevalence of a disease, and incidence rate. Descriptive studies that include follow-up can provide insight into the number of patients that are frequently lost to follow-up. In cases where patients provide data, information can be garnered about change in providers over time. When comparative analysis is performed from registry data, there are limitations to which associations can be drawn, and the importance of confounding must be considered. Although planning of the registry attempts to account for as many confounders as possible, the use of advanced statistical methods—such as stratified analysis, multivariable analysis, propensity scoring, or instrumental variable analysis—may be needed. It is also important in comparative analysis to consider the extent to which bias, especially detection and selection bias, can distort the results. Development of a statistical plan at the onset of analysis to address the primary and secondary objectives of the research question, as well as the overlying hypothesis, drastically simplifies the analytical process and has the best chance of producing a research product with results that can be generalized.

6. Summary

The use of registry data is only going to become more prolific as the cost of randomized control trials increases and patients with increased knowledge about treatment options refuse randomization. In today's era of team science, more collaboration between institutions has allowed registries to be supported at one facility, yet still recognize other institutions and participants. While developing a registry is a huge undertaking, it is not necessary to reinvent the wheel. Well established registries in other areas can provide a base for data collection while giving you access to a structured reporting system and the possibility of collaboration. In our own TOS registry, we allow participation from any other institution. We support other institutions by providing support for patient data collection and supplying data case forms for collection. We also have established electronic portals for both patients and providers to enter data, and we even support entry of data for institutions that do not have resources to extract patient data and enter it into the system. This is all done at no cost to the institution other than support of a resource contact person.

Conflicts of Interest: The author declares no conflicts of interest.

References

1. Merriam-Webster. Registry 2017. Available online: www.merriam-webster.com (accessed on 21 February 2017).
2. Gliklich, R.; Dreyer, N.; Leavy, M. (Eds.) *Registries for Evaluating Patient Outcomes: A User's Guide*, 3rd ed.; Two volumes; Agency for Healthcare Research and Quality: Rockville, MD, USA, 2014. Available online: http://www.effectivehealthcare.ahrq.gov/registries-guide-3.cfm (accessed on 14 February 2017).
3. MacIntyre, K.; Capewell, S.; Stewart, S.; Chalmers, J.W.; Boyd, J.; Finlayson, A.; Redpath, A.; Pell, J.P.; McMurray, J.J. Evidence of improving prognosis in heart failure: Trends in case fatality in 66,547 patients hospitalized between 1986 and 1995. *Circulation* **2000**, *102*, 1126–1131. [CrossRef]
4. Wennberg, D.E.; Lucas, F.L.; Birkmeyer, J.D.; Bredenberg, C.E.; Fisher, E.S. Variation in carotid endarterectomy mortality in the Medicare population: trial hospitals, volume, and patient characteristics. *JAMA* **1998**, *279*, 1278–1281. [CrossRef]
5. Institute of Medicine (US) Roundtable on Value & Science-Driven Health Care. (Ed.) *Learning What Works Best: The Nation's Need for Evidence on Comparative Effectivenss in Health Care*; National Academies Press: Washington, DC, USA, 2007.
6. Research FCCfCE. Report to the President and the Congress. U.S. Department of Health and Human Services, 2009. Available online: http://www.hhs.gov/recovery/programs/cer/cerannualrpt.pdf (accessed on 14 February 2017).
7. LaBresh, K.A.; Gliklich, R.; Liljestrand, J.; Peto, R.; Ellrodt, A.G. Using "get with the guidelines" to improve cardiovascular secondary prevention. *Jt. Comm. J. Qual. Saf.* **2003**, *29*, 539–550. [CrossRef]
8. Charrow, J.; Esplin, J.A.; Gribble, T.J.; Kaplan, P.; Kolodny, E.H.; Pastores, G.M.; Scott, C.R.; Wappner, R.S.; Weinreb, N.J.; Wisch, J.S. Gaucher disease: Recommendations on diagnosis, evaluation, and monitoring. *Arch. Intern. Med.* **1998**, *158*, 1754–1760. [CrossRef]
9. Illig, K.A.; Donahue, D.; Duncan, A.; Freischlag, J.; Gelabert, H.; Johansen, K.; Jordan, S.; Sanders, R.; Thompson, R. Reporting standards of the Society for Vascular Surgery for thoracic outlet syndrome. *J. Vasc. Surg.* **2016**, *64*, e23–e35. [CrossRef]

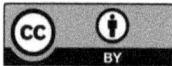

diagnostics

MDPI

Review

Choosing Surgery for Neurogenic TOS: The Roles of Physical Exam, Physical Therapy, and Imaging

David P. Kuwayama [1], Jason R. Lund [2], Charles O. Brantigan [1] and Natalia O. Glebova [1,3,*]

[1] Division of Vascular Surgery and Endovascular Therapy, Department of Surgery, University of Colorado Denver, Denver, CO 80045 USA; david.kuwayama@ucdenver.edu (D.P.K.); cbrantigan@drbrantigan.com (C.O.B.)

[2] Ashbaugh Center for Physical Therapy, Denver, CO 80222, USA; jasonrlund@hotmail.com

[3] Section of Vascular Surgery and Endovascular Therapy, Department of Surgery, University of Colorado Anschutz Medical Campus, 12631 East 17th Ave, Room 5409, Mail Stop C 312, Aurora, CO 80045, USA

* Correspondence: natalia.glebova@ucdenver.edu; Tel.: +1-303-724-2690; Fax: +1-303-724-2693

Received: 23 May 2017; Accepted: 16 June 2017; Published: 23 June 2017

Abstract: Neurogenic thoracic outlet syndrome (nTOS) is characterized by arm and hand pain, paresthesias, and sometimes weakness resulting from compression of the brachial plexus within the thoracic outlet. While it is the most common subtype of TOS, nTOS can be difficult to diagnose. Furthermore, patient selection for surgical treatment can be challenging as symptoms may be vague and ambiguous, and diagnostic studies may be equivocal. Herein, we describe some approaches to aid in identifying patients who would be expected to benefit from surgical intervention for nTOS. We describe the role of physical examination, physical therapy, and imaging in the evaluation and diagnosis of nTOS.

Keywords: neurogenic thoracic outlet syndrome; physical examination; physical therapy; imaging

1. Introduction

Neurogenic thoracic outlet syndrome (nTOS) is a relatively common problem which is frequently not recognized [1]. Some investigators believe that nTOS is overdiagnosed. While they may be right in some circumstances, it is far more likely that nTOS is more commonly underdiagnosed. The diagnosis of nTOS is made by understanding the total clinical picture, and that requires a complete history and physical examination [2]. There is no single test which unequivocally allows the diagnosis to be made in a definitive fashion, but certain imaging modalities may be confirmatory. Symptoms of nTOS are similar to symptoms caused by a wide variety of other conditions. Furthermore, a patient may have multiple coexisting conditions, and the challenge is to identify the etiology of various parts of the symptom complex before making recommendations. These patients look normal in spite of pain and dysfunction. They have often been seen by other physicians, many of whom have decided that the symptoms are psychogenic. The stresses caused by chronic symptoms, coupled with the cursory examinations carried out by some physicians, reinforce the conclusion that the problem is psychogenic. Multiple visits to physicians, who either do not believe nTOS exists or who believe that it is a diagnosis of exclusion, aggravate the emotional problems that these patients experience. Since there are no definitive tests for nTOS, the diagnosis is made by performing complete history and physical examinations to develop an understanding of the total clinical picture. The examining physician needs to understand that TOS is usually neurological and much less commonly vascular.

2. Physical Examination in Evaluation of Neurogenic Thoracic Outlet Syndrome (nTOS)

In this day of increasingly complex testing, the patient is often compartmentalized. In the case of nTOS, patients are referred for a determination of the presence or absence of nTOS. It is important to understand that these complicated patients need to have a comprehensive evaluation, including a thorough review of their records, even if there are so many records that they have to be brought on a flatbed truck. This really needs to be done, even though it takes a significant amount of physician time, with no payment for the physician who performs this service. After record review, these patients need a comprehensive history and physical examination with the goal of finding out what is wrong with the patient as a whole. Guided by the examination, tests may be offered and therapy planned. The key is to remember that nTOS occurs in patients with anatomic abnormalities [3] and to look for these on physical examination.

The typical history of patient with lower brachial plexus nTOS consists of discomfort and pain of varying intensity at the base of the neck [4]. The pain radiates down the arm through the ulnar aspect of the forearm into the hand. These patients have paresthesias affecting the ulnar distribution of the hand. Severe headaches are associated with lower brachial plexus nTOS [4]. They generally start at the base of the skull and radiate over the top of the head. The headaches are usually related to arm use rather than the time of day. In some patients, the pain may radiate into the anterior chest simulating cardiac angina. Sleeve like numbness of the arm awakens him or her at night. This is associated with pain in the upper extremity and numbness and pain which radiate down the arm and into the ulnar innervated areas of the hand. In more advanced cases, weakness of the hand and loss of dexterity of the fingers frequently develops. There may be muscle atrophy and impaired use of the arm without paralysis. Arm extension and elevation typically aggravates the symptoms. Activity during the day the results in misery at night, whereas quiet days lead to more comfortable nights. Symptoms typically occur after exercise rather than during exercise. This is the most common presentation of nTOS. As you examine the patient, look for tenderness of the band spot described below, paresthesias, weakness of elbow extension compared to flexion, weakness of the intrinsic muscles of the hand, and numbness in the ulnar distribution.

The typical patient with upper brachial plexus nTOS presents with the same pain in the neck experienced by the lower brachial plexus patient, but also has pain radiating upward to the ear. These patients may have pain affecting the face and temple and hemicranial headaches. They may complain of a stuffy ear with a negative otologic examination. The pain radiates to the upper pectoral area and laterally through the trapezius muscle and down the outer arm. On physical exam, these patients often have a Tinel's sign radiating into the trapezius and rhomboid muscles. Look for thenar weakness and a Tinel's sign in the neck.

The physical examination starts when the patient is first introduced to the examiner and concludes as the patient walks out of the examination room. The physician needs to figure out what sort of disease the patient has, as well as what sort of patient has the disease. What is the patient's overall state of wellbeing? What does he or she look like from across the room? Is the patient's function limited by nTOS or by another condition? Is stress amplifying the symptoms? Each finding on initial observation often adds focus to further examinations. As much as possible, abnormal findings should be confirmed with another observation or another physical test. Nonphysiological symptoms must be sought. Does he or she have abnormal use of the extremities? Does he or she carry a back pack of large purse? Is that compatible with the symptoms? Are there spontaneous motions of the neck or the extremities observed which do not match the history? Are the symptoms incompatible with the physician's observations? Or are there signs of non physiologic findings, such as breakaway weakness, or contraction of all muscles of the body except the muscle being tested?

At the conclusion of the evaluation it may be best to schedule another appointment. That appointment might be to follow up on any tests ordered. More important than the tests is the opportunity to reexamine the patient to see how consistent the symptoms and findings are over time, which may be difficult if the patient is from out of town. Another important consideration is to determine patient expectations. Caution is advised if the patient has seen many doctors and wants an operation. Additionally, be wary of patients with unrealistic expectations who characterize previous doctors as incompetent. Appropriate patient selection for surgical intervention is key to obtaining excellent outcomes in the treatment of nTOS [5–7].

One must remember that patients with nTOS usually have an underlying structural anomaly with superimposed trauma, and then look for the anomaly [3]. The trauma may have been severe, but more often the trauma is low intensity occupation induced repetitive activity. Compare one arm to the other looking for swelling, atrophy or another source of assymetry. Look for evidence of vasospasm. Unilateral Raynaud's phenomenon suggests a local problem such as nerve impingement. Presence of vasospasm in the other hand could be subclinical and indicate a systemic process. This can be evaluated in the vascular laboratory with a cold immersion test.

Physical examination should be systematic and begin with the neck [8]. Check range of motion of the neck, with or without axial loading or pretend axial loading. If the patient complains of pain on neck rotation, position yourself so that he or she has to rotate the neck see what you are doing. See if the symptoms are present even when he or she thinks you are examining something else. See if axial loading causes more symptoms. If it does, then check rotation again with the examiner's hand on the top of the head but without applying pressure. Try to find the stub of a cervical rib in the posterior aspect of the neck. Palpate the neck musculature for spasm which can cause TOS symptoms by itself. Identify which muscles in particular are in spasm, as that can guide subsequent physical therapy and provides a baseline for follow-up. Check the response to gentle fist percussion of the spine; palpate the spine looking for specific sites of tenderness, such as cervical disks.

Apply gentle pressure to the anterior scalene looking for pain and possibly pain radiating into the arm or paresthesias radiating to the face and ear. Apply gentle pressure to the band spot, a point in the base of the neck anterior to the trapezius where a type 3 band connects to the first rib [3]. Generalized tenderness does not count. Percuss the anterior scalene placed on the stretch and look for radiation from the site of percussion expecting a Tinel's sign up along the cheek, into the eye and into the pectoralis area in the case of upper brachial plexus nTOS. In lower brachial plexus nTOS, numbness from palpation of the band spot radiates down the arm and into the last two digits. Palpate the area where the pectoralis minor inserts to the coracoid process looking for palpable spasm of the pectoralis minor and possibly Tinel's sign radiating into the upper extremity. In the few cases where the pectoralis minor is the culprit, one can often feel the pectoralis minor through the relaxed pectoralis major. In all of these tests, point tenderness rather than generalized tenderness constitutes a positive test.

Examine the shoulders and arms next [8]. Look for evidence of a winged scapula. Palpate the area of the rhomboid major muscle looking for tenderness and spasm. Check the strength of abduction adduction, flexion, and extension of the shoulder looking for evidence of shoulder impingement syndrome, which can often be identified by pain and weakness of external and internal rotation. Palpate the shoulder joint looking for localized tenderness from tendonitis. Look for Raynaud's phenomenon, particularly if it is unilateral. Check for medial and lateral epicondylitis. Check the motor strength of flexion and extension of the elbow and of the wrist. In patients with lower brachial plexus nTOS, there is generally weakness of elbow extension compared to flexion on the involved side. Dorsiflexion of the wrist should be examined as well, as that is a monitor for upper brachial plexus nTOS. Check deep tendon reflexes. Look for Tinel's sign over the ulnar nerve at the elbow and median nerve at the wrist.

The hands are evaluated next. Examine for the possibility of carpal tunnel syndrome by tapping the median nerve at the wrist, checking for atrophy in the thenar eminence in the case of carpal tunnel syndrome, and in the small muscles of the hand in pronounced forms of nTOS. Check the strength of thumb opposition both to the index finger or the little finger. Check for weakness of the intrinsic muscles of the hand using interphalangeal card test and palpation of the hand with fingers spread or held tightly together. Check grip strength and thumb opposition at the same time. Do a sensory examination of the arm using both light touch and light pinprick. Perform Phelan's test which reproduces the patient's symptoms in cases of carpal tunnel syndrome. Phelan's test is performed with the arms at the patient's side and the elbows flexed at 90 degrees. The dorsal surfaces of the hands are placed so that the wrists are flexed 90 degrees. This position is held for 60 s looking for reproduction of the patient's symptoms.

Physical examination maneuvers aimed at specifically evaluating for nTOS should also be performed and include Adson's test and Elevated Arm Stress Test (EAST) [9]. Adson first described his test in 1927 [10]. It is performed with the patient seated with the arms resting on the knees. The patient takes a long deep breath and elevates the chin and turns the head to the affected side. An alteration or obliteration of the radial pulse was considered to be pathonemonic for the scalenus anticus syndrome. Other observers add abduction and external rotation of the arm as part of the positioning. Adson's writings indicate that he was using this test to identify patients who had attachment of the lower anterior scalene muscle to the subclavian artery. It may have had some usefulness in identifying this subset of patients, but it does not apply to the other forms of TOS. In addition, the test is positive as often in normal patients as it is in patients with thoracic outlet syndrome.

The elevated arm exercise test or the elevated arm stress test (EAST) is the most reliable test for the diagnosis of nTOS. It is performed by having the patient put both arms in the 90° abduction external rotation position with the shoulders and elbows in the frontal plane of the chest. The patient is instructed to slowly open and close the hands over the course of 3 min. Normal patients can perform the stress test for 3 min with only mild muscle fatigue and minimal distress. Patients with nTOS, on the other hand, commonly find reproduction of the usual symptoms with an increase in pain in the neck and shoulder. There is aching progressing down the arm, and paresthesias develops in the forearm and the ulnar innervated fingers. Those with arterial compression will develop arm pallor with the arm elevated and reactive hyperemia when it is lowered. Those with venous compression may develop cyanosis and swelling associated with the pain. Many patients with nTOS will be unable to complete this test and will drop the arms after only a brief period of exercise. They recognize symptoms as reproduction of the usual symptoms. Patients who have carpal tunnel syndrome may experience some numbness with this test, but it is from compression of the median nerve and the symptoms will be confined primarily to the first 3 fingers with some radiation up the arm.

One important distinction must be made when evaluating a patient with nTOS. It is possible that a patient with psychosomatic illness as the cause of his or her symptoms is referred for evaluation for nTOS. Diagnosis of psychosomatic illness needs to be made with the same precision as that of nTOS. Frost in 1972 emphasized that these patients should not be characterized as malingering [11]. They are better characterized as having a psychogenic caricature of somatic disability. Their prognosis is good if they do not get an operation. The key concept in evaluation of these patients is to repeat tests of the same function and look for variations in response and disparity between symptoms and physical findings, particularly over time.

3. Physical Therapy in Evaluation of nTOS

An important component of evaluation of patients with potential nTOS is physical therapy (PT). The diagnosis of nTOS can be difficult and often involves multiple examinations and tests to differentiate TOS from other implicating diagnoses [12]. This section describes an effective PT assessment of patients with potential nTOS developed over many years of experience with this patient population. The assessment focuses on a specific evaluation and its contribution to implicating nTOS as causation of symptoms and an important factor for determining surgical candidates.

The subjective history can provide significant clues as to when symptoms are being produced, as well as the instigating or exacerbating factors [9]. The activity that is linked to symptom production can drive the physical exam based on involved anatomy and the effect on the narrow passageways of nerves and blood vessels. The passageways include the scalene triangles, costoclavicular space and the sub pectoral space. Other important pieces of information can be gathered from prior trauma to the clavicle, shoulder pathology affecting scapulothoracic mechanics or cervical pathology. The time of day when symptoms arise can indicate whether there is a tensioning event or a release event. The tension of a nerve produces ischemia and venous pooling around the nerve and it takes 6 h before the return of normal flow [13]. Upon return of normal flow, paresthesia will be present as axons will begin to fire and may explain the release event [14].

nTOS may be difficult to diagnose as traction of the brachial plexus is intermittent, and there may not be constant sensory or motor deficits. Usually, the first signs to present are non-radicular pain and paresthesia. Visual inspection of static posture is noted with regard to head and shoulder position. Movement provides better clues of dysfunction based on what structural mobility occurs or what myofascial tension impacts movement. As an example, abduction of the scapula needs to take place during active arm elevation for proper kinematics. A dyskinetic scapula might wing secondary to poor muscle recruitment of serratus anterior or abnormal tightness in pectoralis minor that attaches to coracoid process of the scapula. Therefore, PT evaluation needs to be dynamic to reveal mechanical dysfunction that may be producing traction and provoking symptoms. This also sets the PT examination apart from what the function of other disciplines in diagnosis of these patients.

The PT physical examination involves mobility tests for provocation or functional movement. Testing of the first rib is the most imperative. A spring test in sitting position can reveal both first rib mobility with end feel as well as pain provocation. The Lindgren test is a very reliable test for an elevated first rib and involves cervical rotation and contralateral side bending. An elevated first rib will prevent available movement of C7. The Roos test and the Cyriax maneuver are both provocation tests that use scapular position for indication based on result. Roos test places the patient in an abducted, retracted and depressed scapular position and involves having the patient open and close their hands for 3 min, increasing vascular demand. A test is considered positive if the symptoms are reproduced. The Cyriax maneuver involves unloading the shoulder girdle with the examiner standing behind the patient and bringing the shoulder girdle into elevation. This test is also held for 3 min and considered positive if tingling is reproduced. When normal flow through a nerve is restored, axons will fire producing paresthesia, so the test is looking for a release event based on scapular position.

Vascular tests include assessment of the radial pulse and placement of the patient in a certain position. Adson's test, which looks for the disappearance of the radial pulse with a patient's arm being passively extended while the patent extends and rotates their head toward the examiner. They are asked to hold their breath while assessing for the disappearance of the radial pulse and can implicate the scalenes. Eden's test involves measuring the radial pulse while the examiner tractions the arm and compresses the clavicle. It can implicate costoclavicular space compression. Wright's test looks specifically at the sub pectoral passageway and involves hyperabduction of the arm to tension the pectoralis minor and subsequent reproduction of symptoms or change in radial pulse.

Specific neural tension tests of the ulnar, median and radial nerve can provide information about sensitivity to mechanical loading [15]. Despite evidence that the roots of C5, C6, and C7 are fixed to transverse processes [16] and will not always be as sensitive and specific in diagnosing nTOS, neural irritation rarely allows for mobility of the nerve without a response. Furthermore, neural mobilization tests can try to differentiate between lesions in the proximal and distal parts of the nerve by changing the pressure at tension points and evaluating the patient's response to the change in tension.

Functional testing involves assessment of the anatomical structures that make up each passageway. Assessment in the cervical spine is also crucial for differentially diagnosing pure cervical pathology versus a residual effect from changing joint mechanics or muscle recruitment. Loading tests such as a Spurling test and unloading tests such as manual traction can provide significant information as to pure cervical related pathology. Assessment of segmental joint mobility can reveal hypo or hypermobility issues at each joint that can then be investigated through their adjacent level relationship or muscle synergistic patterns. Special attention is paid to the cervicothoracic junction as the level where cervical mobility meets thoracic rigidity. Assessment continues down into the thoracic spine measuring both joint position and mobility. Rib articulation with the thoracic spine and spring mobility test can identity dysfunctional structures. Other important joints to assess for mobility are the sternoclavicular and acromioclavicular and their connection to scapular thoracic mobility. Finally, palpation of muscles that form borders of the aforementioned passageways is important to determine length tension as well as provocation, paying special attention to hypertrophy and hypertonia [17]. Comparison with the asymptomatic side can be used for indication of dysfunction.

Once dysfunctions are identified, an appropriate treatment plan can be constructed to influence the narrow passageways through which the neurovascular tissue has become irritated. Objective improvements of these dysfunctions can be measured and compared with overall improvement of the patient's symptoms. As a basis, some objective improvement should occur during a 6-week period of consistent non-operative management. Resolution of symptoms that allow for return to function is the long-term goal. However, those patients who do not make any or enough improvement can become candidates for surgery. The surgical procedure of removing the first rib and resecting the anterior scalene is designed to improve the space the brachial plexus has to descend into the arm. So, for the operation to have an optimal outcome, the patient needs to have had direct or indirect dysfunction of the structure that is common to all passageways where compression or traction can occur—the first rib.

The physical therapist's role in recognizing candidates for whom an operation will produce the best outcome, is based on his or her clinical examination, as well as the candidate's response to the physical therapy treatment program. Non-operative management that has taken place over the 6-week period allows for ongoing assessment of anatomy and changes to the objective findings that treatment has been trying to influence. Treatment involves a comprehensive approach of manual therapy directed at bone or joint position, soft tissue mobilization, and therapeutic exercise focusing on recruitment of stabilization based musculature and inhibition of over-utilized muscles. Protocols specific to the underlying pathology of nTOS should be utilized [6,18]. Postural training should be included in non-operative management [19]. Physical therapy may be successful in treating the symptoms of nTOS such that an operation is not required [19,21–23]. Continual access to the patient also allows for assessment of compliance to a home exercise program and changes to body mechanics and postural recommendations during function. As treatment progresses, the physical therapist looks for improvement in objective findings to match at least some symptom improvement. When non-operative treatment has been effective with objective measures, but symptoms respond and revert without linear progression, it is appropriate to recommend these patients for surgical consideration.

4. The Role of Imaging in Diagnosis of nTOS

Optimal imaging for diagnosis of neurogenic thoracic outlet syndrome (nTOS) remains controversial. Because the underlying pathophysiology is presumed to be bony, muscular or fibrous compression of brachial plexus fibers, imaging tests revolve around modalities that can either identify these structures or assess the function of nerve fibers traversing the thoracic outlet [3]. Conversely, contrast imaging focused on evaluation of the subclavian artery or vein, while useful for evaluation of arterial (aTOS) or venous TOS (vTOS), are typically only suggestive of associated neural compression.

4.1. Plain Films

In patients with suspected nTOS, the recommended initial screening test remains plain antero-posterior radiograms of either the cervical spine or chest. Plain films are widely available, low cost, and result in only minimal radiation exposure. A plain film evaluated by a trained interpreter can efficiently screen for a wide variety of potentially relevant bony anomalies, such as incomplete or complete cervical ribs, elongated C7 transverse processes, anomalous first ribs, and anomalous clavicles.

A retrospective review by Weber [22] of preoperative imaging in 400 surgically treated TOS patients revealed that of the 219 with neurogenic TOS, 23% had a cervical rib and 10% had another bony anomaly (first rib, clavicle) [23]. Cervical rib presence was significantly higher in nTOS patients than those with other forms of TOS (23% vs. 16%, $p < 0.05$), while there was no significant difference between the groups with respect to other bony anomalies (10% vs. 7%, $p = 0.20$). In comparison, large population based studies of routine chest films have identified cervical ribs in only 1% of healthy subjects.

While identification of a bony anomaly, particularly a cervical rib, on plain film may be suggestive of a possible associated nerve compression syndrome, no compelling data exists regarding sensitivity, specificity or accuracy of this finding when compared either to operative findings or to emerging gold standard imaging tests such as CT or MRI. In particular, the absence of a bony anomaly on plain film should not be interpreted as lessening the likelihood of thoracic outlet compression syndrome.

4.2. Computed Tomography

Computed tomography (CT) possesses numerous major advantages over plain radiography for evaluation of the thoracic outlet [24,25]. Multi-detector CT technology has improved over the years to permit high-resolution (1 mm cut or less) imaging, and computer processing power now enables rapid 3D reconstruction of images by even non-radiologists (Figure 1). Synchronous administration of timed contrast boluses permits evaluation of the arteries and veins, and has become the gold standard for evaluation of the vascular structures in the thoracic outlet. However, although skilled interpreters may be able to identify brachial plexus structures on CT, nerves are not as well visualized on CT as on MRI.

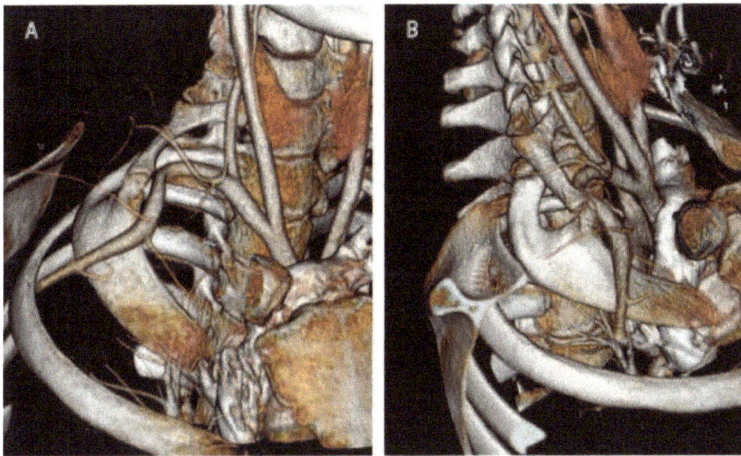

Figure 1. 3D reconstruction of computed tomography (CT) arteriography, demonstrating a right-sided cervical rib fused to a broadened first thoracic rib, with anterior displacement of the subclavian artery. (**A**) antero-posterior view; (**B**) oblique view.

A crucial aspect to CT imaging for evaluation of TOS is the use of provocative positioning. Images are first obtained with the arms in neutral position at the sides; subsequently, images are obtained with the arms raised above the head in an attempt to elicit narrowing of the thoracic outlet. Mastumura performed CT arteriography and CT venography in 10 healthy patients, both with and without provocative positioning [24]. Importantly, he found moderate to severe venous compression to be essentially universal with arm elevation, but found that arterial compression in healthy volunteers was either absent or minimal. As such, provocative CT findings of venous compression may reflect normal physiology and should not be considered pathognomonic for nTOS, but findings of arterial compression or arterial aneurysm formation should be taken more seriously.

Remy Jardin et al. performed standard and provocative CT angiography in 79 patients with symptomatic TOS, at least 80% of whom had a neurogenic component, and evaluated changes in the morphologies of the three compartments of the thoracic outlet (interscalene triangle, costoclavicular space and subcoracoid tunnel) [26]. Although he identified a variety of changes in bony and arterial positioning with arm elevation, the most significant finding was a statistically significant reduction in the average maximum distance between the clavicle and first rib (34% reduction in females; 24% reduction in males), contributing to significant compression of the neurovascular bundle.

4.3. Magnetic Resonance Imaging

Magnetic resonance imaging (MRI) is gaining importance in the evaluation of the thoracic outlet. In addition to bone and vessels, MRI permits evaluation of the cervical nerve roots and brachial plexus cords; normal and abnormal muscular structures; and presence of abnormal fibrous bands. Just as with CT, images may be obtained with provocative positioning, although the narrowness of the imaging bore may make arm elevation prohibitive for some body types.

Both Yildizgören et al. and Baumer et al. have reported on the MRI-assisted discovery of fibrous bands in the thoracic outlet causing brachial plexopathies, and Muellner et al. reported on the MRI-assisted discovery of an aberrant subclavius posticus muscle narrowing the costoclavicular space [27–29]. None of these abnormalities would have been identifiable on CT images or plain radiogram, demonstrating the significant advantage of MRI over CT for visualization of soft tissue abnormalities in the thoracic outlet.

Evolution of MRI technology has yielded particular benefits for visualization of nerves, a potential major advance in the diagnosis of neurogenic TOS. As strength of closed MRI magnets has increased to 3T, novel sequencing techniques (e.g., Short Tau Inversion Recovery (STIR), Spectral Attenuated Inversion Recovery (SPAIR)), steady state with 3D volumetric acquisition) have permitted vastly improved visualization of nerves, a technology termed MR neurography (MRN). The addition of diffusion tensor imaging (DTI) to standard MRN sequences may even permit visualization of individual nerve fascicles. Such techniques may permit direct imaging of nerve compression or impingement by bony, muscular, or fibrous structures [30]. In classic nTOS, MRN may be able to directly visualize anomalies of the lower brachial plexus cords, such as compression, flattening, or neural and peri-neural inflammation. Such findings may support the contention that anatomic correction of the underlying compression syndrome would be therapeutic; conversely, the absence of any visible lower cord anomalies may be grounds for further diagnostic workup into other potential syndromes.

Beyond its importance in visualization of the thoracic outlet and its components, MRI also permits detailed evaluation of surrounding structures whose dysfunction may mimic the symptoms of nTOS, including evaluation of the cervical spine for assessment of spinal stenosis or cervical disc disease, and evaluation of the shoulder for intrinsic joint or tendon disease.

4.4. Positional MRI

Several investigators have documented the feasibility and added diagnostic utility of MRI with provocative positioning. Nevertheless, positional MRI remains rarely used in clinical practice, and its applicability has not been proven in sizable clinical series.

Demondion et al. first reported positional MRI of the thoracic outlet in a proof-of-concept study using 5 cadavers and 12 healthy volunteers [31]. With a 1.5T magnet, he obtained T1 weighted spin-echo sequences first with the arms alongside the body, then with the arms hyperabducted at 135 degrees. In all scans, the various components of the thoracic outlet were well visualized (interscalene triangle, prescalene space, costoclavicular space and retropectoralis minor space). Sagittal sequences were most useful, as they enabled visualization of the nervous and vascular structures in cross section as they traversed the relevant spaces.

In a larger follow up study, Demondion et al. reported on 35 healthy volunteers and 54 symptomatic patients with TOS who underwent 1.5T MRI imaging with arms in both neutral and hyperabducted positioning [32]. Notably, vascular and nervous compression was visualized only with the arms abducted, reinforcing the importance of provocative positioning. The quality of imaging was sufficient to enable quantitative assessment of bony, muscular, and fibrous components of the thoracic outlet (e.g., minimum costoclavicular distance, subclavius muscle thickness). It was also able to demonstrate specific sites of compression from fibrous bands, underlining the fundamental advantage of a discriminating soft-tissue imaging technique such as MRI over CT.

Smedby et al. performed similar testing on 10 healthy volunteers and 7 patients, but used an open MRI scanner with a 0.5T magnet [33]. The use of an open scanner enabled provocative patient positioning without the associated difficulties of fitting into a narrow bore. Sagittal 3D SPGR sequences were obtained and were of sufficient quality to permit visualization of brachial plexus compression and narrowing of the costoclavicular space

4.5. Other Diagnostic Imaging

While MRI and CT have proven to be the most widespread and useful forms of imaging for TOS, application of other imaging modalities, including duplex ultrasound and formal angiography, has been described in the literature. In general, these have proven to be of limited utility for neurogenic TOS.

Demondion et al. attempted to use duplex ultrasound to map the brachial plexus in healthy volunteers and obtained satisfactory visualization in 10 of 12 subjects [34]. Imaging quality was best when using high-frequency linear probes transmitting from 10 to 13 MHz. Of note, the costoclavicular space (a common site of compression in neurogenic TOS) was not directly visualizable due to shadowing artifact, and deeper structures such as the eighth cervical and first thoracic nerve roots were difficult to visualize. He concluded that ultrasound imaging was of potential value for purposes of regional anesthetic administration, but less so for diagnosis of bony compression syndromes. He also found that the quality of imaging was highly dependent on both sonographer technique and patient body habitus.

Simon et al. was able to diagnose a case of neurogenic TOS secondary to a fibrous band extending from an elongated C7 transverse process. Imaging in this case was aided by the fact that compression was not due to an overlying bony structure, but rather, a fibrous band, minimizing shadow artifact [35]. The ultrasound diagnosis was subsequently confirmed with MR neurography and intraoperative findings. Thus, while occasional cases of nTOS may be identifiable with ultrasound, the inability to directly visualize the costoclavicular space remains a major limitation of this technique.

Although resolution of CT and MR imaging has steadily improved, intraluminal defects in arteries and veins remain best visualized on formal angiography (arteriography and venography). These tests permit excellent definition of thrombus, dissection flaps, and other intravascular anomalies. Additionally, provocative positioning with contrast administration may elicit evidence of positional compression syndromes (Scherrer et al.) [36]. However, these tests provide no visualization of neurologic structures and are, therefore, of no value for purely neurogenic TOS. Because of its invasive nature, diagnostic angiography for nTOS is only warranted when clinical suspicion exists for a combined thoracic outlet syndrome with both neurogenic and vascular components, and in situations of diagnostic dilemma unsolvable by CT or MRI imaging.

4.6. Electrodiagnosis

In addition to imaging techniques for visualization of thoracic outlet compression, electrodiagnostic evaluation of the innervation of an affected arm may provide corroborating evidence of brachial plexus compression or damage. It may be of particular use in situations in which imaging has been unable to demonstrate compression, but clinical suspicion for thoracic outlet related neuropathy remains high.

The typical electrodiagnostic findings in nTOS involve lower brachial plexopathy affecting the lower trunk, C8 and T1 nerve roots [37]. On sensory testing, the most commonly affected nerve is the medial antebrachial cutaneous (MABC) nerve, a cutaneous branch of the medial cord that receives most of its fibers from the T1 nerve root and innervates the skin overlying the distal biceps and medial forearm. On motor testing, the most commonly weakened muscle group is the abductor pollicis brevis, a contributor to thumb abduction and a major muscular component of the thenar eminence. This muscle is innervated by the recurrent branch of the median nerve, which receives many of its fibers from the C8 and T1 nerve roots. Atrophy of this muscle can lead to wasting of the thenar eminence noticeable on physical exam.

Tsao et al. reported on pre-operative electrodiagnostic findings in 32 patients with surgically verified nTOS and confirmed that a T1-focused examination, combining MABC and median nerve testing, was abnormal in 89% of study subjects, while response combinations focused on C8 fibers were less sensitive [38]. This finding of a T1 > C8 axonal loss phenomenon is in contrast to most other kinds of lower brachial plexopathies, which more often affect C8 fibers greater than T1 fibers (e.g., post-median sternotomy). As such, careful performance of electrodiagnostic studies including nerve conduction and needle electrode examination may help discriminate between nTOS and other forms of neurologic injury.

4.7. Interventional Imaging

For both diagnostic and therapeutic purposes, some practitioners advocate percutaneous neuromuscular blockade of the anterior scalene, middle scalene, pectoralis minor and subclavius muscles [39]. By inducing transient or long-lasting paralysis of these muscles, the interscalene triangle and costoclavicular space widen. Relief of symptoms with successful blockade may therefore be highly suggestive or confirmatory of nTOS.

Attempts at anesthetizing or chemodenervating these muscles based upon surface landmarks alone may lead to accidental somatic block or sympathetic block in up to 10% of patients. Consequently, numerous imaging modalities have been used to help guide muscle blockade, including ultrasound, fluoroscopy, CT, and needle electromyography [40]. Jordan et al. retrospectively reviewed 245 thoracic outlet chemodenervation procedures using electromyography for confirmation of needle tip localization, 77 of which used adjunctive ultrasound and 168 of which used adjunctive fluoroscopy [41]. Patients were evaluated for procedural success and for complications including dysphagia, dyshponia, pneumothorax, or undesired muscle weakness. Overall complication rates were less than 2%, and median duration of clinical benefit was 4.7 months. Mashayekh et al. reported on 106 patients undergoing 146 scalene injections using CT guidance. In all cases, needle tip localization was satisfactory [42]. No major complications occurred, although 11% reported minor complications such as needle site pain, temporary brachial plexus block, undesired muscle weakness, dysphagia and Horner sign.

It should be noted that reliance on positivity of muscular blockade for diagnosis of nTOS is controversial. Although many cases of nerve compression may be relieved with muscular relaxation, other forms of nerve compression (e.g., compression by a fibrous band) may prove refractory. As such, it would be inappropriate to interpret failure to respond to muscular blockade as ruling out the possibility of nTOS.

5. Conclusions

Neurogenic TOS is fundamentally an anatomic compression syndrome. As such, the diagnosis is most readily supported by either radiographic imaging of visibly compressed brachial plexus structures or electrodiagnostic findings consistent with sequelae of intermittent compression. Nevertheless, imaging modalities, like any test, remain susceptible to type I and II errors. Some practitioners express concern that overly strict imaging or diagnostic criteria for nTOS may lead to under-diagnosis and under-treatment. Conversely, others believe that visualized compression in the costoclavicular or retropectoral spaces with provocative positioning may reflect normal physiology, thereby leading to over-diagnosis and over-treatment. Therefore, while advances in imaging technology have provided practitioners with a wealth of new information, the formal diagnosis of neurogenic TOS remains firmly rooted in other aspects of evaluation, notably the clinical history and physical exam.

Managing and treating TOS can be frustrating and rewarding. A complete history and physical examination are required to make an accurate diagnosis. Expert physical therapy assessment is integral in helping to establish the diagnosis and identify patients who will benefit from operative intervention. Imaging is helpful in ruling out other conditions and confirming the diagnosis. With appropriately selected patients, excellent outcomes are achievable for this sometimes difficult-to-manage condition. Younger patients with shorter duration of symptoms and fewer narcotics used enjoy better results in the long-term follow up of patients surgically treated for nTOS [6,43]. Patients with chronic pain syndromes, smoking, age $\geq$ 40 years, and opioid use have less favorable outcomes [44]. Patients who are on chronic opioids are challenging to diagnose, and unless physical exam and imaging findings are clear and convincing, operative treatment should probably be avoided. Patients who have had a prolonged history of multiple diagnoses and interventions for upper extremity symptoms may also be poor candidates for surgical treatment. Patients with presumptive nTOS often have antecedent history of accidental injury, and may present within the workers' compensation or disability system. The associated disability may cloud the accuracy of the diagnosis and compensation status correlates with poor outcomes after surgical intervention [45]. It behooves the surgeon to consider that, while in general well-tolerated, operative treatment of nTOS is associated with several risks including injury to the subclavian artery or vein, brachial plexus, or phrenic nerve. Correct diagnosis and careful patient selection are key to successful treatment of patients with this often misdiagnosed condition.

Conflicts of Interest: The authors declare no conflict of interest.

References

1. Freischlag, J.; Orion, K. Understanding thoracic outlet syndrome. *Scientifica* **2014**, *2014*, 248163. [CrossRef] [PubMed]
2. Kuhn, J.E.; Lebus, G.F.; Bible, J.E. Thoracic Outlet Syndrome. *J. Am. Acad. Orthop. Surg.* **2015**, *23*, 222–232. [CrossRef] [PubMed]
3. Roos, D.B. Congenital anomalies associated with thoracic outlet syndrome. Anatomy, symptoms, diagnosis, and treatment. *Am. J. Surg.* **1976**, *132*, 771–778. [CrossRef]
4. Sanders, R.J.; Hammond, S.L.; Rao, N.M. Diagnosis of thoracic outlet syndrome. *J. Vasc. Surg.* **2007**, *46*, 601–604. [CrossRef] [PubMed]
5. Colli, B.O.; Carlotti, C.G.; Assirati, J.A.; Marques, W. Neurogenic thoracic outlet syndromes: A comparison of true and nonspecific syndromes after surgical treatment. *Surg. Neurol.* **2006**, *65*, 262–271. [CrossRef] [PubMed]
6. Orlando, M.S.; Likes, K.C.; Mirza, S.; Cao, Y.; Cohen, A.; Lum, Y.W.; Reifsnyder, T.; Freischlag, J.A. A Decade of Excellent Outcomes after Surgical Intervention in 538 Patients with Thoracic Outlet Syndrome. *J. Am. Coll. Surg.* **2015**, *220*, 934–939. [CrossRef] [PubMed]
7. Chandra, V.; Olcott, C.; Lee, J.T. Early results of a highly selective algorithm for surgery on patients with neurogenic thoracic outlet syndrome. *J. Vasc. Surg.* **2011**, *54*, 1698–1705. [CrossRef] [PubMed]
8. Hoppenfeld, S. *Physical Examination of the Spine and Extremities*; Appleton and Lang: Norwalk, CT, USA, 1976.
9. Brantigan, C.O.; Roos, D.B. Diagnosing thoracic outlet syndrome. *Hand Clin.* **2004**, *20*, 27–36. [CrossRef]
10. Adson, A.W. Surgical treatment for symptoms produced by cervical ribs and the scalenus anticus muscle. *Surg. Gynecol. Obstet.* **1947**, *85*, 687–700. [PubMed]
11. Frost, H.M. Diagnosing musculoskeletal disability of psychogenic origin in orthopaedic practice. *Clin. Orthop. Relat. Res.* **1972**, *82*, 108–122. [CrossRef] [PubMed]
12. Sheth, R.N.; Belzberg, A.J. Diagnosis and treatment of thoracic outlet syndrome. *Neurosurg. Clin. N. Am.* **2001**, *12*, 295–309. [PubMed]
13. Kwan, M.K.; Woo, S.L. Biomechanical properties of peripheral nerve. In *Operative Nerve Repair and Reconstruction*; Gelberman, R., Ed.; J.B. Lippincott Company: Philadelphia, PA, USA, 1991; pp. 47–54.
14. Lundborg, G. Ischemic nerve injury. Experimental studies on intraneural microvascular pathophysiology and nerve function in a limb subjected to temporary circulatory arrest. *Scand. J. Plast. Reconstr. Surg. Suppl.* **1970**, *6*, 3–113. [PubMed]
15. Coppieters, M.W.; Stappaerts, K.H.; Everaert, D.G.; Staes, F.F. Addition of test components during neurodynamic testing: Effect on range of motion and sensory responses. *J. Orthop. Sports Phys. Ther.* **2001**, *31*, 226–235. [CrossRef] [PubMed]

16. Leishout, G.B. Cervical Spondylosis. In *Brain*; Brain, W., Lord, J., Eds.; Heinemann: London, UK, 1967.
17. Sanders, R.J.; Jackson, C.G.; Banchero, N.; Pearce, W.H. Scalene muscle abnormalities in traumatic thoracic outlet syndrome. *Am. J. Surg.* **1990**, *159*, 231–236. [CrossRef]
18. Orlando, M.S.; Likes, K.C.; Freischlag, J.A. Physical Therapy in the Management of Patients with Neurogenic Thoracic Outlet Syndrome. *J. Am. Coll. Surg.* **2015**, *221*, 778–779. [CrossRef] [PubMed]
19. Novak, C.B. Conservative management of thoracic outlet syndrome. *Semin. Thorac. Cardiovasc. Surg.* **1996**, *8*, 201–207. [PubMed]
20. Novak, C.B.; Collins, E.D.; Mackinnon, S.E.; Louis, S. Outcome Following Conservative Management of Thoracic Outlet Syndrome Materials and Methods. *J. Hand Surg.* **1995**, *20*, 542–548. [CrossRef]
21. Wilbourn, A.J.; Porter, J.M. Neurogenic thoracic outlet syndrome: Surgical versus conservative therapy. *J. Vasc. Surg.* **1992**, *15*, 880–882. [CrossRef]
22. Watson, L.A.; Pizzari, T.; Balster, S. Thoracic outlet syndrome Part 2: Conservative management of thoracic outlet. *Man. Ther.* **2010**, *15*, 305–314. [CrossRef] [PubMed]
23. Weber, A.E.; Criado, E. Relevance of Bone Anomalies in Patients with Thoracic Outlet Syndrome. *Ann. Vasc. Surg.* **2014**, *28*, 924–932. [CrossRef] [PubMed]
24. Matsumura, J.S.; Rilling, W.S.; Pearce, W.H.; Nemcek, A.A.; Vogelzang, R.L.; Yao, J.S. Helical computed tomography of the normal thoracic outlet. *J. Vasc. Surg.* **1997**, *26*, 776–783. [CrossRef]
25. Remy-Jardin, M.; Doyen, J.; Remy, J.; Artaud, D.; Fribourg, M.; Duhamel, A. Functional anatomy of the thoracic outlet: Evaluation with spiral CT. *Radiology* **1997**, *205*, 843–851. [CrossRef] [PubMed]
26. Remy-Jardin, M.; Remy, J.; Masson, P.; Bonnel, F.; Debatselier, P.; Vinckier, L.; Duhamel, A. Helical CT Angiography of Thoracic Outlet Syndrome. *Am. J. Roentgenol.* **2000**, *174*, 1667–1674. [CrossRef] [PubMed]
27. Baumer, P.; Kele, H.; Kretschmer, T.; Koenig, R.; Pedro, M.; Bendszus, M.; Pham, M. Thoracic outlet syndrome in 3T MR neurography—Fibrous bands causing discernible lesions of the lower brachial plexus. *Eur. Radiol.* **2014**, *24*, 756–761. [CrossRef] [PubMed]
28. Muellner, J.; Kaelin-Lang, A.; Pfeiffer, O.; El-Koussy, M.M. Neurogenic thoracic outlet syndrome due to subclavius posticus muscle with dynamic brachial plexus compression: A case report. *BMC Res. Notes* **2015**, *8*, 351. [CrossRef] [PubMed]
29. Yildizgören, M.T.; Ekiz, T.; Kara, M.; Yörübulut, M.; Özçakar, L. Magnetic resonance imaging of a fibrous band causing true neurogenic thoracic outlet syndrome. *Am. J. Phys. Med. Rehabil.* **2014**, *93*, 732–733. [CrossRef] [PubMed]
30. Magill, S.T.; Brus-Ramer, M.; Weinstein, P.R.; Chin, C.T.; Jacques, L. Neurogenic thoracic outlet syndrome: Current diagnostic criteria and advances in MRI diagnostics. *Neurosurg. Focus* **2015**. [CrossRef] [PubMed]
31. Demondion, X.; Boutry, N.; Drizenko, A.; Paul, C.; Francke, J.P.; Cotten, A. Thoracic outlet: anatomic correlation with MR imaging. *Am. J. Roentgenol.* **2000**, *175*, 417–422. [CrossRef] [PubMed]
32. Demondion, X.; Bacqueville, E.; Paul, C.; Duquesnoy, B.; Hachulla, E.; Cotten, A. Thoracic outlet: Assessment with MR imaging in asymptomatic and symptomatic populations. *Radiology* **2003**, *227*, 461–468. [CrossRef] [PubMed]
33. Smedby, O.; Rostad, H.; Klaastad, O.; Lilleås, F.; Tillung, T.; Fosse, E. Functional imaging of the thoracic outlet syndrome in an open MR scanner. *Eur. Radiol.* **2000**, *10*, 597–600. [CrossRef] [PubMed]
34. Demondion, X.; Herbinet, P.; Boutry, N.; Fontaine, C.; Francke, J.-P.; Cotten, A. Sonographic mapping of the normal brachial plexus. *Am. J. Neuroradiol.* **2003**, *24*, 1303–1309. [PubMed]
35. Simon, N.G.; Ralph, J.W.; Chin, C.; Kliot, M. Sonographic diagnosis of true neurogenic thoracic outlet syndrome. *Neurology* **2013**, *81*, 1965. [CrossRef] [PubMed]
36. Scherrer, A.; Roy, P.; Fontaine, A. The compression syndrome: A revaluation of the value of postural angiography (author's transl). *J. Radiol.* **1979**, *60*, 417–422. [PubMed]
37. Seror, P. Medial antebrachial cutaneous nerve conduction study, a new tool to demonstrate mild lower brachial plexus lesions. A report of 16 cases. *Clin. Neurophysiol.* **2004**, *115*, 2316–2322. [CrossRef] [PubMed]
38. Tsao, B.E.; Ferrante, M.A.; Wilbourn, A.J.; Shields, R.W. Electrodiagnostic features of true neurogenic thoracic outlet syndrome. *Muscle Nerve* **2014**, *49*, 724–727. [CrossRef] [PubMed]
39. Jordan, S.E.; Machleder, H.I. Diagnosis of thoracic outlet syndrome using electrophysiologically guided anterior scalene blocks. *Ann. Vasc. Surg.* **1998**, *12*, 260–264. [CrossRef] [PubMed]

40. Torriani, M.; Gupta, R.; Donahue, D.M. Sonographically guided anesthetic injection of anterior scalene muscle for investigation of neurogenic thoracic outlet syndrome. *Skelet. Radiol.* **2009**, *38*, 1083–1087. [CrossRef] [PubMed]

41. Jordan, S.E.; Ahn, S.S.; Gelabert, H.A. Combining ultrasonography and electromyography for botulinum chemodenervation treatment of thoracic outlet syndrome: Comparison with fluoroscopy and electromyography guidance. *Pain Physician* **2007**, *10*, 541–546. [PubMed]

42. Mashayekh, A.; Christo, P.J.; Yousem, D.M.; Pillai, J.J. CT-Guided Injection of the Anterior and Middle Scalene Muscles: Technique and Complications. *Am. J. Neuroradiol.* **2011**, *32*, 495–500. [CrossRef] [PubMed]

43. Likes, K.C.; Orlando, M.S.; Salditch, Q.; Mirza, S.; Cohen, A.; Reifsnyder, T.; Lum, Y.W.; Freischlag, J.A. Lessons Learned in the Surgical Treatment of Neurogenic Thoracic Outlet Syndrome Over 10 Years. *Vasc. Endovasc. Surg.* **2015**, *49*, 8–11. [CrossRef] [PubMed]

44. Rochlin, D.H.; Gilson, M.M.; Likes, K.C.; Graf, E.; Ford, N.; Christo, P.J.; Freischlag, J.A. Quality-of-life scores in neurogenic thoracic outlet syndrome patients undergoing first rib resection and scalenectomy. *J. Vasc. Surg.* **2013**, *57*, 436–443. [CrossRef] [PubMed]

45. Harris, I.; Mulford, J.; Solomon, M.; van Gelder, J.M.; Young, J. Association Between Compensation Status and Outcome After Surgery. *JAMA* **2005**, *293*, 1644. [CrossRef] [PubMed]

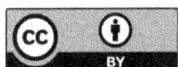

diagnostics

MDPI

Article

Ultrasonographic Diagnosis of Thoracic Outlet Syndrome Secondary to Brachial Plexus Piercing Variation

Vanessa Leonhard [1], Gregory Caldwell [1], Mei Goh [2], Sean Reeder [1] and Heather F. Smith [3,4,*]

[1]   Department of Osteopathic Manipulative Medicine, Arizona College of Osteopathic Medicine, Midwestern University, Glendale, AZ 85308, USA; vleonhard26@midwestern.edu (V.L.); gcaldwell36@midwestern.edu (G.C.); SReede@midwestern.edu (S.R.)
[2]   Arizona College of Osteopathic Medicine, Midwestern University, Glendale, AZ 85308, USA; mgoh24@midwestern.edu
[3]   Department of Anatomy, Midwestern University, Glendale, AZ 85308, USA
[4]   School of Human Evolution and Social Change, Arizona State University, Tempe, AZ 85287, USA
*   Correspondence: hsmith@midwestern.edu; Tel.: +1-623-572-3726; Fax: +1-623-572-3679

Received: 28 April 2017; Accepted: 29 June 2017; Published: 4 July 2017

Abstract: Structural variations of the thoracic outlet create a unique risk for neurogenic thoracic outlet syndrome (nTOS) that is difficult to diagnose clinically. Common anatomical variations in brachial plexus (BP) branching were recently discovered in which portions of the proximal plexus pierce the anterior scalene. This results in possible impingement of BP nerves within the muscle belly and, therefore, predisposition for nTOS. We hypothesized that some cases of disputed nTOS result from these BP branching variants. We tested the association between BP piercing and nTOS symptoms, and evaluated the capability of ultrasonographic identification of patients with clinically relevant variations. Eighty-two cadaveric necks were first dissected to assess BP variation frequency. In 62.1%, C5, superior trunk, or superior + middle trunks pierced the anterior scalene. Subsequently, 22 student subjects underwent screening with detailed questionnaires, provocative tests, and BP ultrasonography. Twenty-one percent demonstrated atypical BP branching anatomy on ultrasound; of these, 50% reported symptoms consistent with nTOS, significantly higher than subjects with classic BP anatomy (14%). This group, categorized as a typical TOS, would be missed by provocative testing alone. The addition of ultrasonography to nTOS diagnosis, especially for patients with BP branching variation, would allow clinicians to visualize and identify atypical patient anatomy.

Keywords: anatomical variation; brachial plexus; superior trunk; middle trunk; anterior scalene muscle; neurogenic thoracic outlet syndrome; ultrasound; provocative testing

1. Introduction

Neurogenic thoracic outlet syndrome (nTOS) is a neurologic impingement syndrome that is notoriously difficult to diagnose in the clinical setting [1,2]. There are vascular and neurogenic forms of thoracic outlet syndrome (TOS), with nTOS being the most common and comprising over 90% of cases [3]. The arterial type, affecting the subclavian artery, is more concretely diagnosable by traditional provocative tests [1], as these directly evaluate the radial pulse. Adson's [4], Wright's, and Costoclavicular tests utilize the classic relationship of the subclavian artery and the branches of the brachial plexus to identify specific sites of neurovascular impingement (Table 1). These tests diagnose compression at three distinct sites: within the interscalene space, deep to the pectoralis minor tendon, and between the first rib and clavicle. Adson's test evaluates the passage of the brachial plexus trunks and subclavian artery as they pass through the interscalene space between the anterior and middle scalene muscles and relies on change in radial pulse due to compression of the subclavian artery between those muscles [4].

Table 1. Summary of standard provocative tests typically used to diagnose thoracic outlet syndrome and to rule out other upper extremity neurogenic conditions.

Provocative Test	Condition Tested	Description	Positive Test
TOS Tests			
Adson's Test	Thoracic outlet syndrome (TOS)	Tests for compression of subclavian artery between anterior and middle scalene muscles. Monitor radial pulse with abduction, extension, and external rotation of upper extremity, and the head turned toward the affected side and then away.	Marked reduction of radial pulse or reproduction of symptoms
Costoclavicular Test	Thoracic outlet syndrome (TOS)	Tests for compression of subclavian artery between clavicle and first rib. Monitor radial pulse with patient forcefully hyper-retracting their scapulae.	Reduction of radial pulse
Hyperabduction/Wright Test	Thoracic outlet syndrome (TOS)	Tests for compression of subclavian artery by pectoralis minor muscle. Monitor radial pulse while holding the affected arm in a position of hyperabduction coupled with hyperextension.	Reproduction of symptoms or reduction of radial pulse
Rule-out Tests			
Carpal Compression Test	Carpal Tunnel Syndrome	Tests for impingement of the median nerve as it courses deep to the transverse carpal ligament. With wrist supinated, compress the carpal ligament.	Numbness and tingling within the median nerve distribution
Modified Spurling's Test	Cervical root compression	Tests for cervical root compression at the cervical foramina. Patient's head extended, ipsilaterally rotated, and ipsilaterally tilted with axial loading.	Reproduction of symptoms beyond shoulder blade

However, recent studies have determined that in individuals with brachial plexus branching variants [5–7], the nerve branches may be impinged within the anterior scalene muscle belly, while the subclavian artery travels unencumbered. These structural variants undermine traditional provocative testing by violating the assumption of concomitant impingement of the neurologic and arterial structures. Cadaveric study has uncovered a significant percentage of variation of the brachial plexus trunks at this level [5–7]. In the most prevalent variation, the superior piercing variation, the superior trunk (or its components: the anterior rami of C5 and C6) pierces the anterior scalene muscle. A multiple piercing variant was observed as well, in which the superior and middle trunks both pass independently through the anterior scalene muscle [7]. Together, these piercing variants have been found in with up to 48% of individuals deviating from the classic anatomical arrangement [7]. In patients with a structural variation in which portions of the brachial plexus course through the anterior scalene, this test would be falsely negative. These structures create increased diagnostic difficulty as the current diagnostic standard in the primary care setting relies on identical passage of the artery and plexus through this space.

TOS most commonly presents with neurological symptoms of pain and paresthesias, recorded in 98–100% of TOS patients (e.g., [8–10]). Symptoms are primarily located in the proximal arm (88%), shoulder (88%), and all five digits (58%) [3]. These nonspecific findings are associated with numerous forms of pathology in the upper extremity and the cervical region [11–14]. Similarly, the current definitions of TOS vary among clinicians. One study determined that surgeons are 100 times more likely to diagnose TOS than neurologists [15]. In general, current diagnostic criteria typically require that the provocative tests cause vascular change at the radial artery, regardless of symptoms. Disputed, or non-specific TOS is quite common, occurring when patients present with TOS-like symptoms, but do not meet the currently accepted diagnostic standards and, therefore, lack a definitive explanation for their symptoms (e.g., [16]). Individuals with variations from classic anatomical relationships, such as the superior piercing variation, are likely to present in this manner and remain without clear diagnosis or treatment strategy. To achieve more comprehensive diagnosis and plan of care, ultrasonography may offer a means to visualize the anatomy of the thoracic outlet, identify clinically relevant variations, and provide a distinct diagnosis for these patients.

Previous studies into the efficacy of provocative testing indicated that up to 60% of asymptomatic patients experienced vascular compromise during testing, a diagnostic false positive for TOS [17–19]. Considering the high prevalence of variation within the brachial plexus trunks, and associated lack of vascular change, the Adson's test also has a high propensity for false negatives, up to 10%. One explanation for these results may be that a subset of patients presenting with nTOS symptoms, may be variant in the relationships of the thoracic outlet structures. Ultrasound imaging may be able to visualize these brachial plexus variants, therefore providing a diagnosis for those who would otherwise be missed by provocative testing.

Recently, new sets of criteria for diagnosing TOS have been proposed [20–22]. The Consortium for Outcomes Research and Education on Thoracic Outlet Syndrome proposed a preliminary set of detailed diagnostic TOS criteria [20,22]. This comprehensive list is an invaluable resource. However, while the study acknowledges that scalene muscular variation may exist, the implication is that such variation is rare and "too small to be detected by standard imaging tests, such as plain X-rays, CT or MRI scanning" and can, therefore, only be assessed at the time of surgery [22]. A second set of updated TOS reporting standards were recently published by the Society for Vascular Surgery [21] which include: symptoms of pathology at the thoracic outlet, symptoms of nerve compression, the absence of other pathology potentially explaining the symptoms, and a positive scalene muscle injection test. While useful, these standards do not account for common structural variation at the thoracic outlet. The criteria presume that "the brachial plexus and subclavian artery traverse the same spaces" [21] (p. e25). Therefore, patients with brachial plexus branching variants would lack the first diagnostic criterion because they have no pathology present at the thoracic outlet, only a common anatomical variation. Another potential limitation of this set of standards is that it requires the use of scalene muscle injections, which may not be accessible to a primary care physician in the clinic. Recently, electrodiagnostic methods have been developed which can result in more objective neurological findings regarding TOS (e.g., [23]). However, for the average primary care physician, this technology may not be available in the clinic and, thus, the use of these techniques is primarily relegated to specialists.

Given the recent discovery that piercing variants in the brachial plexus are quite common [5–7], and may predispose these individuals to nTOS, this study seeks to empirically evaluate the proposed association between brachial plexus piercing variants and nTOS symptoms. We also aim to determine the applicability of ultrasonography (US) for increasing the efficacy of clinical diagnosis over traditional provocative testing alone, especially for cases of nTOS secondary to BP variation.

2. Materials and Methods

2.1. Cadaveric Data

The cadaveric investigation assessed proximal brachial plexus branching variation in 95 cadaveric brachial plexus specimens (44 male, 51 female) from the gross anatomy teaching laboratories at Midwestern University. Cadavers were obtained for teaching purposes from the National Body

Donation Program (St. Louis, MO, USA). The neck and shoulder of each cadaver were dissected bilaterally following *Grant's Dissector* 16th ed. [24] to thoroughly reveal the brachial plexus. The inferior and lateral borders of the anterior scalene muscle were defined, and the position of the roots, trunks, and cords of the brachial plexus in relation to the scalene muscles was determined and documented. For each cadaveric specimen, the type(s) of brachial plexus branching variation and sidedness of each variant was recorded. Each specimen was evaluated by two members of the research team to confirm the assessment, and photo-documented for future confirmation. *t*-tests were then performed in SPSS 19 (IBM Corp., Chicago, IL, USA) to assess whether significant differences existed in the frequency of brachial plexus variants between the sexes.

2.2. Ultrasonography

Twenty-two volunteer student subjects were recruited from Midwestern University in Glendale, AZ, USA. Screening began with a comprehensive questionnaire covering pertinent past medical history, trauma history, and symptoms of neurovascular pathology in the upper extremity. Subjects were then tested using standard nTOS provocative testing, including Adson's, Costoclavicular, and Hyperabduction/Wright tests (Table 1). Additional tests to rule out other upper extremity neurogenic conditions were also utilized, including Carpal Compression and Modified Spurling's tests (Table 1). Any changes in radial arterial pulse or reproduction of symptoms were noted. The protocol for this study was approved by Midwestern University's Institutional Review Board (IRB AZ#885, 9 March 2016).

Following completion of provocative testing, participants underwent ultrasound (US) study of the lateral neck using a Sonoscape S8 portable ultrasound unit. Starting with the US probe in the supraclavicular fossa, imaging was completed up to the angle of the mandible in both neutral and Adson's test position bilaterally. A visual scan was conducted to identify the three hypoechoic trunks with a hyperechoic fascial separation from the anterior and middle scalene muscles. A lack of visible hyperechoic fascia between the anterior scalene and any of the trunks indicated a brachial plexus piercing variant. The branching pattern of the proximal brachial plexus, and the relationship of the trunks to the scalene muscles were documented bilaterally. Still images and video capture were used to record the anatomy for future verification. Researchers conducting US were blind to the results of the questionnaire and provocative testing. Ultrasound results were confirmed with a board certified radiologist.

To determine whether statistically significant correlations exist between reported TOS symptoms, brachial plexus branching variants (as identified by ultrasound) and provocative test results, a series of statistical analyses were conducted in SPSS 19 (IBM Corp.). Brachial plexus branching (ultrasound) results were coded as: piercing versus classic anatomy. Provocative test results were coded as separate variables for: any positive pulse or symptom reproduction during test, pulse response, and symptoms reproduced. Due to the bilaterally asymmetrical nature of brachial plexus branching, the left and right sides for each subject were considered separately. Bivariate correlation analyses were then performed between TOS symptoms and: brachial plexus variation, and each of the provocative test results. Partial correlation analyses were subsequently conducted between TOS symptoms and provocative test results while controlling for brachial plexus variation.

3. Results

3.1. Cadaveric Results

In the cadaveric sample (n = 95 plexi), brachial plexus branching variants were extremely common (Tables 2 and S1). Only 32 brachial plexi (33.7%) were found to possess the "classic" anatomical pattern in which all three trunks of the brachial plexus course through the interscalene triangle (Figure 1). In the sample, 63 variations from the classic anatomical pattern were observed (Table 2, Figure 2B,C), such that 66.3% of the sample did not display the classic relationship between the scalene musculature and proximal brachial plexus. These variations can be classified into four categories: superior piercing (54.7%), multiple piercing (4.2%), C5 piercing (3.2%), and C5 anterior variant (3.4%). In each variant, one or more components of the brachial plexus course(s) in a position of relative vulnerability where it is more likely to become impinged. The most common clinically-relevant variants are depicted in Figure 2. The variant anatomy occurred more frequently in male cadavers than in females (74.5% vs. 56.8%); however, the *t*-test indicated that these differences between the sexes did not reach the statistical threshold for significance ($t = -1.83$, $p = 0.07$).

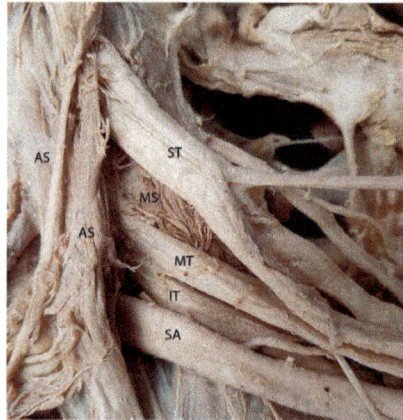

Figure 1. Cadaveric photo illustrating the classic anatomical relationship between the scalene musculature and the trunks of the brachial plexus. In this arrangement, the superior, middle, and inferior trunks of the brachial plexus all course between the anterior and middle scalene muscle, through the interscalene gap. AS = anterior scalene; IT = inferior trunk; MS = middle scalene; MT = middle trunk; SA = subclavian artery; ST = superior trunk.

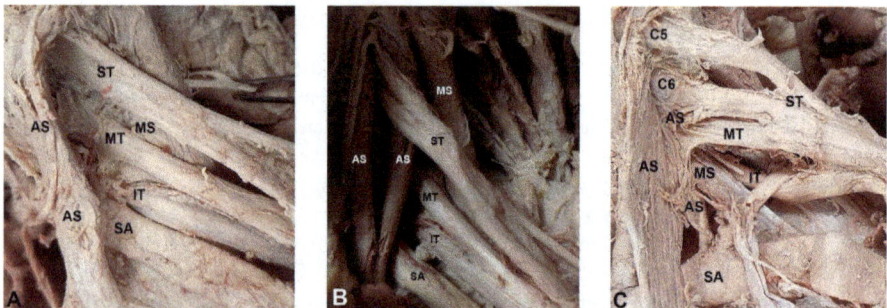

Figure 2. Anatomical relationships between the proximal brachial plexus and scalene musculature identified in the cadaveric component of the present study: (**A**) classic anatomical relationship between the brachial plexus and anterior scalene muscle. Superior, middle, and inferior trunks of the brachial plexus travel with the subclavian artery through the interscalene gap, between the anterior and middle scalene muscles; and (**B**) the superior piercing variant. The superior trunk of the brachial plexus pierces the anterior scalene muscle; and (**C**) the multiple piercing variant. The superior and middle trunks of the brachial plexus pierce the anterior scalene muscle. AS = anterior scalene; C5 = anterior ramus of C5; C6 = anterior ramus of C6; IT = inferior trunk; MS = middle scalene; MT = middle trunk; SA = subclavian artery; ST = superior trunk.

Table 2. Summary of cadaveric dissection results: quantification of anatomical variants in the relationship between the proximal brachial plexus and the scalene musculature.

Gender of Subjects	Classic Anatomy	C5 Anterior	Superior Piercing	Multiple Piercing	C5 Piercing
Male	13	2	29	4	3
Female	19	2	23	0	0
Total (%)	32 (33.7%)	4 (4.2%)	52 (52.7%)	4 (4.2%)	3 (3.2%)

3.2. Ultrasonographic Results

In the ultrasonographic screening sample, 79.5% of the sample was found to possess classic brachial plexus anatomy (Figure 3), while a total of nine brachial plexus branching variants were identified (20.5%) (Tables 3 and S2). Eight of these were classified as piercing variants, in which portions of the brachial plexus coursed through the anterior scalene muscle (18.2%). The most common variation was the superior piercing variant ($n = 4$; 9.1%) (Figure 4), followed by the multiple piercing variant ($n = 3$; 6.8%) (Figure 5), and C5 piercing variant ($n = 1$; 2.3%) (Figure 6). There was also one example of a non-piercing anterior variant (2.3%) (Figure 7).

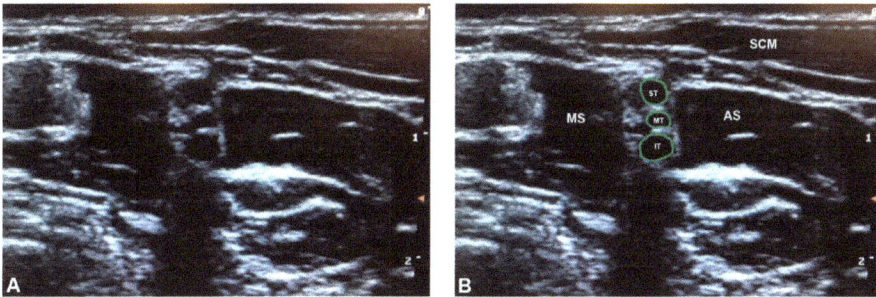

Figure 3. The classic brachial plexus anatomy identified on ultrasound: (**A**) unlabeled; and (**B**) labeled. Note that the superior, middle, and inferior trunks are clearly separated from the anterior and middle scalene muscles by hyperechoic fascial planes. AS = anterior scalene; IT = inferior trunk; MS = middle scalene; MT = middle trunk; SCM = sternocleidomastoid; ST = superior trunk. The green outlines demarcate the trunks of the brachial plexus.

Table 3. Brachial plexus variation in the screening sample, as identified by ultrasonographic evaluation.

Brachial Plexus Pattern	Frequency in Sample	% Symptomatic
Classic Anatomy	35; 79.5%	5; 13.9%
C5 Anterior Variant	1; 2.3%	0; 0%
Piercing Variants: Total	8; 18.2%	4; 50%
C5 Piercing Variant	1; 2.3%	1; 100%
Superior Piercing Variant	4; 9.1%	2; 50%
Multiple Piercing Variant	3; 6.8%	1; 33%

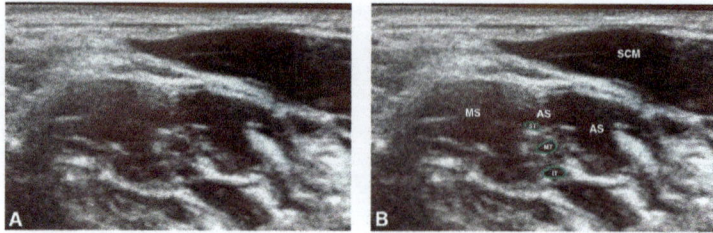

Figure 4. The superior piercing variant, the most common brachial plexus variant, identified using ultrasonography in the present study: (**A**) unlabeled; and (**B**) labeled. Note that the superior trunk is not separated from the anterior scalene in this condition, visible as a lack of hyperechoic fascia. AS = anterior scalene; IT = inferior trunk; MS = middle scalene; MT = middle trunk; SCM = sternocleidomastoid; ST = superior trunk. The green outlines demarcate the trunks of the brachial plexus.

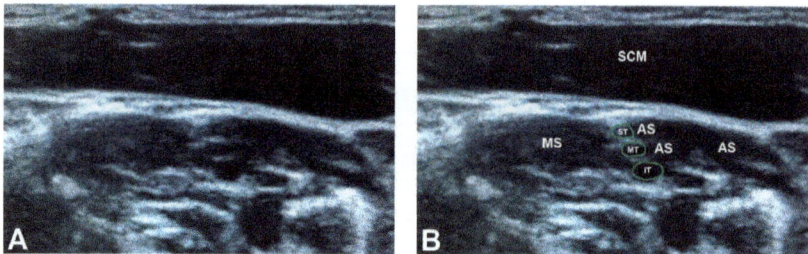

Figure 5. The multiple piercing variant, identified using ultrasonography in the present study: (**A**) unlabeled; and (**B**) labeled. Note that the superior and middle trunks are not separated from the anterior scalene in this condition, visible as a lack of hyperechoic fascia. AS = anterior scalene; C5 = anterior ramus of C5; C6 = anterior ramus of C6; IT = inferior trunk; MS = middle scalene; MT=middle trunk; SCM = sternocleidomastoid; ST= superior trunk. The green outlines demarcate the trunks and roots of the brachial plexus.

Of the eight instances of piercing variants, four were found in association with nTOS symptoms (50%), in contrast to five symptomatic instances in the 38 normal plexuses (13.9%) (Figure 8). The correlation analysis revealed a statistically significant correlation between brachial plexus piercing variants and nTOS symptoms ($r = 0.345$, $p = 0.022$). We classified these patients as presenting with atypical TOS, in which the nTOS symptoms are caused by impingement of the brachial plexus within the anterior scalene muscle belly, rather than in the interscalene gap. The other four atypical brachial plexus variant individuals may still be at increased risk for TOS based upon their anatomy; however, at the time of this study, they were asymptomatic. The sensitivity, specificity, positive predictive values and negative predictive value were determined to be 44%, 88.6%, 50%, and 86.1%. These values were determined using patient reported symptoms as a surrogate gold standard. The criteria for included symptoms was based upon common characteristics of nTOS described in the current literature. This surrogate was selected because it represents the patient population that would present for diagnosis and treatment in a clinical setting.

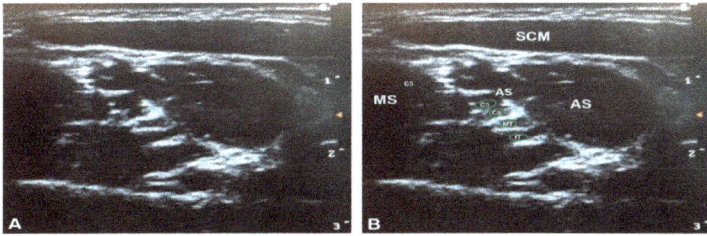

Figure 6. The C5 piercing variant, identified using ultrasonography in the present study: (**A**) unlabeled; and (**B**) labeled. Note that the C5 anterior ramus is not separated from the anterior scalene in this condition, visible as a lack of hyperechoic fascia. AS =anterior scalene; C5 = anterior ramus of C5; C6 = anterior ramus of C6; IT = inferior trunk; MS = middle scalene; MT = middle trunk; SCM = sternocleidomastoid; ST = superior trunk. The green outlines demarcate the trunks and roots of the brachial plexus.

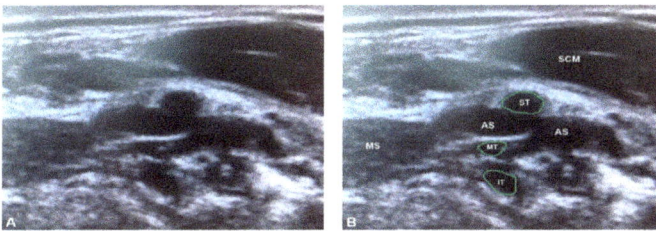

Figure 7. The anterior variant, identified using ultrasonography in the present study: (**A**) unlabeled; and (**B**) labeled. Note that the superior trunk courses superficial to the anterior scalene muscle in this condition. AS = anterior scalene; IT = inferior trunk; MS = middle scalene; MT = middle trunk; SCM = sternocleidomastoid; ST = superior trunk. The green outlines demarcate the trunks of the brachial plexus.

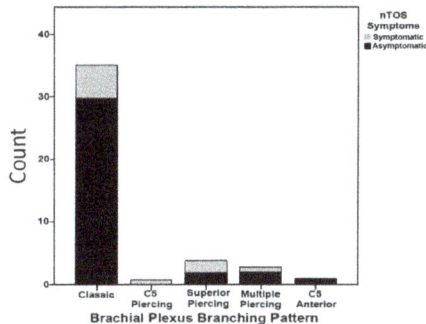

Figure 8. Frequency of brachial plexus branching patterns identified via ultrasonography in the screening portion of this study, and association with reported symptoms consistent with neurogenic thoracic outlet syndrome (nTOS). Symptomatic subjects are indicated in grey, while asymptomatic subjects are indicated in black. The percentages of symptomatic subjects are significantly higher in the piercing variant categories than in the normal sample of subjects with classic brachial plexus anatomy.

Across the entire sample, there were nine total instances of reported symptoms consistent with nTOS (20.5%), which is consistent with the presentations common to TOS as documented in previous studies [9,10]. Given that the student population is predicted to be at higher risk for neurogenic symptoms due to hypertonicity of the cervical musculature, a minor increase in cases was expected in this study. Within the full clinically symptomatic group, three subjects (33.3%) had positive Adson's tests, while two had positive Wright tests (22.2%) (Table 4). These individuals represent the subset of Typical TOS in which the compression occurs between hypertonic anterior and middle scalene muscles.

Table 4. Summary of findings of provocative testing and their association with self-reported neurogenic thoracic outlet syndrome (nTOS) symptoms across the entire screening sample.

Provacative Test Results and nTOS Symptoms	Adson's Test	Costoclavicular Test	Hyperabduction /Wright Test
Positive test and reported nTOS symptomatic	3/16 (18.8%)	2/8 (25.0%)	3/13 (23.1%)
Negative test and reported nTOS asymptomatic	22/28 (78.6%)	29/36 (80.6%)	25/31 (80.6%)

Within the group of participants who denied symptoms on questionnaire ($n = 35$), the provocative tests demonstrated substantial potential for false positives. There were seventeen instances in which a positive result was found for at least one of the three provocative tests without a history of symptoms (48.6% false positives). Of these 17 overall positives, 13 were positive Adson's tests (Figure 9). The correlation analyses revealed no statistically significant correlations between nTOS symptoms and any of the provocative tests (for all results, pulse, and symptoms). The partial correlation analysis controlling for brachial plexus variation also revealed no significant correlation between nTOS symptoms and the provocative tests.

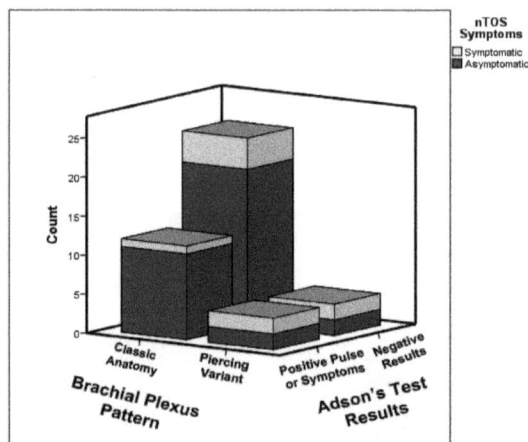

Figure 9. Summary of brachial plexus pattern and Adson's Test results as associated with nTOS symptoms across the full screening sample. Symptomatic subjects are indicated in light grey, while asymptomatic subjects are indicated in dark grey. The percentage of individuals with nTOS symptoms was significantly higher among the brachial plexus piercing variant subjects (50%) than in the subjects with classic brachial plexus anatomy (13.9%), but rates of correct diagnostic identification with Adson's Test were slightly lower (50% in piercing variants vs. 61.1% in classic).

4. Discussion

4.1. Anatomical Variation Observed

The findings from this study support the hypothesis that some cases of disputed TOS may result from brachial plexus variations in which the roots or trunks of the plexus course through the anterior scalene muscle belly, becoming impinged. This phenomenon is similar to piriformis syndrome, which can result from fibers of the sciatic nerve traveling through the piriformis muscle belly leading to impingement. We have determined that individuals with these structural variations in the thoracic outlet present with nTOS symptoms at a significantly higher rate than the general population, but that such anomalies are easily identified using ultrasonography.

Overall, nine of 44 of our student subject brachial plexuses were documented to have variant branching on US imaging, with the majority being the superior piercing variant. Four subjects presented with TOS secondary to a brachial plexus piercing variant. In each of these, the superior trunk or both the superior and middle trunks pierce the anterior scalene muscle (Figures 2 and 4). Clinically, the superior piercing variant would cause neurologic symptoms in the C5 and C6 dermatomal distribution of the lateral arm, thumb, and second digit. Specifically, weakness and sensory deficits in the first two digits, and diminished reflexes of the biceps brachii and brachioradialis muscles [25–28]. The multiple piercing variant (Figure 2C) would result in more extensive neurogenic issues, corresponding with symptoms along the C5, C6, and C7 dermatomes, affecting the first through third digits of the hand. The clinical consequences could also include additional muscle weakness or decreased reflexes in the triceps brachii muscle [26–28].

One screening study participant and two cadavers were found to have *anterior variants*, with the superior trunk passing superficial to the anterior scalene muscle (Figure 6). This variation is less common than the piercing variants, and would not cause numbness or paresthesia in the hands or arms, but could render the nerve vulnerable to compression by forces such as those exerted by purses or backpacks. Impingement of the superior trunk, one of its proximal branches or the supraclavicular nerve is commonly known as pack palsy, which results from pressure on the shoulder girdle and is common in military personnel and hikers [29].

4.2. Diagnosis and Treatment of Thoracic Outlet Syndrome (TOS)

In the general population, primarily typical TOS has been clinically studied and is frequently diagnosed by vascular change with provocative testing. When a patient presents to a clinician with Atypical TOS, there is a potential for premature dismissal of TOS in the differential diagnosis. The diagnosis becomes increasingly elusive because the initial presentation and history of Atypical TOS correlate with other forms of neurologic impingement. Without proper identification of the etiology, the patient may not receive the most efficacious treatment. Based on the results of this study, with nearly half of reported TOS cases originating from variant anatomy which cannot be identified using provocative testing, it can be concluded that US may be a useful adjunct in clinical diagnosis. Ultrasonography is uniquely able to visualize variations and provide clinicians with an understanding of individual anatomy. By combining other diagnostic modalities, such as provocative tests, which can identify hypertonicity impingement, with US, clinicians would have the ability to visualize the structural composition of the neck and shoulder. The inclusion of such knowledge provides a higher level of diagnostic acuity when screening patients presenting with nonspecific TOS symptoms. Scalene blocks are another commonly performed diagnostic modality for nTOS, and can be less equivocal than provocative testing (e.g., [30]). However, these blocks may not be feasible in the primary care setting, and can leave patients with 2–36 h of residual discomfort or inconvenience following the procedure. US, on the other hand, is painless, rapid, and inexpensive, and can be easily implemented as part of a broader diagnostic approach. Due to the varied and complicated nature of nTOS presentation, it is often necessary for clinicians to apply multiple diagnostic modalities before ultimately arriving at a diagnosis. US can serve as an additional resource in the diagnostic toolkit of clinicians, especially in the primary care setting.

Utilizing this diagnostic approach it is also possible to tailor treatment to the individual's unique anatomy. Treatment methods targeting either the first rib or scalene musculature would be complicated by the nerve branches entwined in the anterior scalene muscle belly. Surgical removal of rib 1 would likely not relieve the symptoms of compression around a more laterally placed trunk. A scalenectomy could place the piercing trunks in danger of damage unless appropriately identified [31]. Scalene botulinum toxin injection could be effective, so US could be applied to preselect patients with piercing variants for this treatment. For patients with one of the piercing variations, we propose a rational plan of osteopathic manipulative treatment (OMT) care and/or physical therapy consisting of indirect treatment modalities and the avoidance of direct techniques, based upon the potential for further impingement of the nerve within the muscle belly. This was evidenced in one subject suffering from atypical TOS resulting from a piercing variant [32]. In this case, the patient experienced optimal relief from her symptoms only when indirect treatment techniques were employed, reporting a significant improvement of her symptoms [32]. This patient also had improvement of her concurrent anxiety after gaining a more thorough understanding of her diagnosis with the US imaging.

5. Conclusions

Structural variations of the thoracic outlet, especially common brachial plexus branching variants, create a unique risk for neurogenic TOS that is difficult to diagnose clinically. Ultrasound is a reliable means of diagnosing this etiology when combined with provocative testing and patient history. Identification of these structural variants is crucial for developing an appropriate treatment plan, as certain types of current treatment modalities would be ineffective, or even exacerbate symptoms in patients with these variants.

Supplementary Materials: Supplementary materials can be found at www.mdpi.com/2075-4418/07/3/40/s1.

Acknowledgments: Funding for this research was provided by Midwestern University. The authors would like to thank Katherine Worden, Riley Landreth, Richard Geshel, and Sabina Kumar for their contributions and insight on an earlier version of this study. We thank Brent Adrian for helpful advice regarding figures, and Randall Nydam for his gracious accommodation with the ultrasound unit. Heather F. Smith would also like to thank Gwenneth P. Smith, PT, for insightful discussion regarding nerve compression, neural tension, and treatment modalities, which greatly improved this paper.

Author Contributions: Vanessa Leonhard and Gregory Caldwell developed the project concept and contributed to data collection, data summary review, abstract composition, and manuscript construction; Mei Goh contributed to abstract composition and manuscript review; Sean Reeder contributed to concept development, interpretation of results, and manuscript preparation; and Heather F. Smith developed the project concept, conducted statistical analysis and evaluation, and contributed to data collection, data summary review, and manuscript construction.

Conflicts of Interest: The authors declare no conflict of interest.

References

1. Hooper, T.L.; Denton, J.; McGalliard, M.K.; Brismée, J.M.; Sizer, P.S. Thoracic outlet syndrome: A controversial clinical condition. Part 1: Anatomy, and clinical examination/diagnosis. *J. Man. Manip. Ther.* **2010**, *18*, 74–83. [CrossRef] [PubMed]

2. Kuhn, J.E.; Lebus, G.F.; Bible, J.E. Thoracic Outlet Syndrome. *J. Am. Acad. Orthop. Surg.* **2015**, *23*, 222–232. [CrossRef] [PubMed]

3. Sanders, R.J.; Hammond, S.L.; Rao, N.M. Diagnosis of thoracic outlet syndrome. *J. Vasc. Surg.* **2007**, *64*, 601–604. [CrossRef] [PubMed]

4. Adson, A.W.; Coffey, J.R. Cervical rib: A method of anterior approach for relief of symptoms by division of the scalenus anticus. *Ann. Surg.* **1927**, *85*, 839–857. [CrossRef] [PubMed]

5. Harry, W.G.; Bennett, J.D.; Guha, S.C. Scalene muscles and the brachial plexus: Anatomical variations and their clinical significance. *Clin. Anat.* **1997**, *10*, 250–252. [CrossRef]

6. Sakamoto, Y. Spatial relationships between the morphologies and innervations of the scalene and anterior vertebral muscles. *Ann. Anat.* **2012**, *194*, 381–388. [CrossRef] [PubMed]

7. Leonhard, V.; Smith, R.; Caldwell, G.; Smith, H.F. Anatomical variations in the brachial plexus roots: Implications for diagnosis of neurogenic thoracic outlet syndrome. *Ann. Anat.* **2016**, *206*, 21–26. [CrossRef] [PubMed]

8. Peet, R.M.; Henriksen, J.D.; Anderson, T.P.; Martin, G.M. Thoracic-outlet syndrome: Evaluation of a therapeutic exercise program. *Proc. Staff Meet. Mayo Clin.* **1956**, *31*, 281–287. [PubMed]

9.   Stanton, P.E.; McClusky, D.A.; Richardson, H.D.; Lamis, P.A. Thoracic Outlet Syndrome: A Comprehensive Evaluation. *South. Med. J.* **1978**, *71*, 1070–1073. [CrossRef] [PubMed]

10. Sanders, R.J.; Hammond, S.L.; Rao, N.M. Thoracic outlet syndrome: A review. *Neurologist* **2008**, *14*, 365–373. [CrossRef] [PubMed]

11. Warrens, A.N.; Heaton, J.M. Thoracic outlet compression syndrome: The lack of reliability of its clinical assessment. *Ann. R. Coll. Surg. Engl.* **1987**, *69*, 203–204. [PubMed]

12. Jordan, S.E.; Machleder, H.I. Diagnosis of thoracic outlet syndrome using electrophysiologically guided anterior scalene blocks. *Ann. Vasc. Surg.* **1998**, *12*, 260–264. [CrossRef] [PubMed]

13. Sucher, B.M. Thoracic outlet syndrome—Postural type: Ultrasound imaging of pectoralis minor and brachial plexus abnormalities. *PM&R* **2012**, *4*, 65–72.

14. Strakowski, J.A. *Ultrasound Evaluation of Focal Neuropathies, Correlation with Electrodiagnosis*; Demos Medical: New York, NY, USA, 2014; pp. 127–158.

15. Campbell, W.W.; Landau, M.E. Controversial entrapment neuropathies. *Neurosurg. Clin. N. Am.* **2008**, *19*, 597–608. [CrossRef] [PubMed]

16. Lindgren, K.A.; Leino, E.; Manninen, H. Cervical rotation lateral flexion test in brachialgia. *Arch. Phys. Med. Rehabil.* **1992**, *73*, 735–737. [PubMed]

17. Gergoudis, R.; Barnes, R.W. Thoracic outlet arterial compression: Prevalence in normal persons. *Angiology* **1980**, *31*, 538–541. [CrossRef] [PubMed]

18. Nord, K.M.; Kapoor, P.; Fisher, J.; Thomas, G.; Sundaram, A.; Scott, K.; Kothari, M.J. False positive rate of thoracic outlet syndrome diagnostic maneuvers. *Electromyogr. Clin. Neurophysiol.* **2008**, *48*, 67–74. [PubMed]

19. Sadeghi-Azandaryani, M.; Bürklein, D.; Ozimek, A.; Geiger, C.; Mendl, N.; Steckmeier, B.; Heyn, J. Thoracic Outlet Syndrome: Do we have clinical tests as a predictor for the outcome after surgery? *Eur. J. Med. Res.* **2009**, *14*, 443–446. [CrossRef] [PubMed]

20. Illig, K.A. *Thoracic Outlet Syndrome*; Thompson, R.W., Freischlag, J.A., Donahue, D.M., Jordan, S.E., Edgelow, P.I., Eds.; Springer Science and Business Media: New York, NY, USA, 2014.

21. Illig, K.A.; Donohue, D.; Duncan, A.; Freischlag, J.; Gelabert, H.; Johansen, K.; Jordan, S.; Sanders, R.; Thompson, R. Reporting standards of the 271 Society for Vascular Surgery for thoracic outlet syndrome. *J. Vasc. Surg.* **2016**, *64*, e23–e35. [CrossRef] [PubMed]

22. TOS Consortium. Available online: http://tos.wustl.edu/What-is-TOS/TOS-Consortium (accessed on 3 April 2017).

23. Tsao, B.E.; Ferrante, M.A.; Wilbourn, A.J.; Shields, R.W. Electrodiagnostic features of true neurogenic thoracic outlet syndrome. *Muscle Nerve* **2014**, *49*, 724–727. [CrossRef] [PubMed]

24. Detton, A.J. *Grant's Dissector*, 16th ed.; Wolters Kluwer: Philadelphia, PA, USA, 2016.

25. Roos, D.B. The place for scalenectomy and first-rib resection in thoracic outlet syndrome. *Surgery* **1982**, *92*, 1077–1085. [PubMed]

26. Wood, V.E.; Ellison, D.W. Results of upper plexus thoracic outlet syndrome operation. *Ann. Thorac. Surg.* **1994**, *58*, 458–461. [CrossRef]

27. Urschel, H.C.; Razzuk, M.A. Neurovascular compression in the thoracic outlet. *Ann. Surg.* **1998**, *228*, 609–617. [CrossRef] [PubMed]

28. Matsuyama, J.S.; Okuchi, K.; Goda, K. Upper plexus thoracic outlet syndrome. *Neurol. Med. Chir.* **2002**, *42*, 237–241. [CrossRef]

29. Corkill, G.; Lieberman, J.S.; Taylor, R.G. Pack palsy in backpackers. *West. J. Med.* **1980**, *132*, 569–572. [PubMed]

30. Braun, R.M.; Shah, K.N.; Rechnic, M.; Doehr, S.; Woods, N. Quantitative assessments of scalene muscle block for the diagnosis of suspected thoracic outlet syndrome. *J. Hand Surg.* **2015**, *40*, 2255–2261. [CrossRef] [PubMed]

31. Povlsen, B.; Hansson, T.; Povlsen, S.D. Treatment for thoracic outlet syndrome. *Cochrane Data Syst. Rev.* **2014**. [CrossRef]
32. Leonhard, V.; Landreth, R.; Caldwell, G.; Smith, H.F.; Geshel, R. A case of neurogenic thoracic outlet syndrome secondary to anatomical variation in the brachial plexus identified by ultrasonography. Poster Presented at 2016 American Academy of Osteopathy Annual Convocation, Orlando, FL, USA, 18 March 2016.

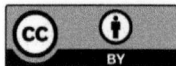

diagnostics

MDPI

Review

Pectoralis Minor Syndrome: Subclavicular Brachial Plexus Compression

Richard J. Sanders * and Stephen J. Annest

The Department of Surgery, University of Colorado Health Science Center, Aurora,
Colorado and Presbyterian-St. Lukes Hospital, Denver, CO 80202, USA; stephenannest@comcast.net
* Correspondence: rsanders@ecentral.com; Tel.: +1-303-756-5877; Fax: +1-303-539-0737

Received: 12 May 2017; Accepted: 30 June 2017; Published: 28 July 2017

Abstract: The diagnosis of brachial plexus compression—either neurogenic thoracic outlet syndrome (NTOS) or neurogenic pectoralis minor syndrome (NPMS)—is based on old fashioned history and physical examination. Tests, such as scalene muscle and pectoralis minor muscle blocks are employed to confirm a diagnosis suspected on clinical findings. Electrodiagnostic studies can confirm a diagnosis of nerve compression, but cannot establish it. This is not a diagnosis of exclusion; the differential and associated diagnoses of upper extremity pain are always considered. Also discussed is conservative and surgical treatment options.

Keywords: neurogenic thoracic outlet syndrome; NTOS; thoracic outlet syndrome; TOS; pectoralis minor syndrome; PMS; neurogenic pectoralis minor syndrome; NPMS; numbness and tingling; pain in neck and arm; occipital headache

1. Introduction

Brachial plexus compression occurs either above the clavicle in the thoracic outlet area or below the clavicle under the pectoralis minor muscle (PMM). Because the symptoms of the two conditions are similar, the history and physical examination is the same for neurogenic thoracic outlet syndrome (NTOS) and neurogenic pectoralis minor syndrome (NPMS). The combination of paresthesia in the hand and pain in the arm should raise the question of brachial plexus involvement. Detailed history and physical examination are needed to determine whether brachial plexus compression is above the clavicle in the thoracic outlet area or below the clavicle, beneath the pectoralis minor muscle. In many patients, the two conditions coexist. No diagnostic test is pathognomonic for NTOS or for NPMS. Evaluation should begin with the clinical picture [1].

2. Anatomy

The anatomy of the structures around the brachial plexus, both above and below the clavicle, are seen in Figure 1. The scalene triangle lies in the thoracic outlet area; the pectoralis minor muscle lies immediately below the clavicle, above the brachial plexus and axillary vessels.

Three anatomical spaces can be identified through which the neurovascular bundle passes. The bundle consists of the triad of brachial plexus, subclavian artery, and subclavian vein. The bundle passes from above the clavicle in the scalene triangle, directly under the clavicle in the costoclavicular space, and below the clavicle under the pectoralis minor muscle (Figure 2 [2]).

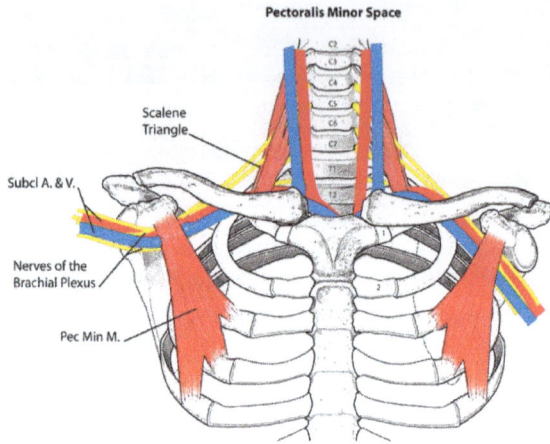

Figure 1. The anatomy of thoracic outlet and pectoralis minor areas. The scalene triangle is above the clavicle. Between the anterior and middle scalene muscles are the five nerve roots and trunks of the brachial plexus and the subclavian artery. The subclavian vein runs anterior to the triangle. Below the clavicle the axillary artery and vein lie immediately under the pectoralis minor muscle. The cords and branches of the brachial plexus usually surround the axillary artery. Figure 1 is reprinted with permission from Sanders R.J. and Haug C.E.: Thoracic outlet syndrome: A common sequela of neck injuries; Lippincott: Philadelphia, PA, USA [2]. Abreviations: Subcl A.&V., subclavian artery and vein; Pec Min M., pectoralis minor muscle.

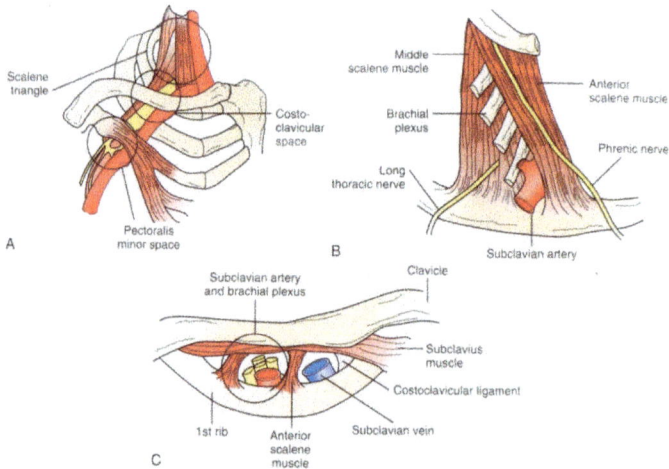

Figure 2. The three anatomical spaces for the neurovascular bundle. (**A**) Pectoralis minor space; (**B**) Scalene triangle; (**C**) costoclavicular space. Reprinted with permission from Sanders R.J. and Haug C.E.: Thoracic outlet syndrome: A common sequela of neck injuries; Lippincott: Philadelphia, PA, USA [2].

3. History

History should begin with a list of current symptoms. Here, current refers to symptoms that have been present for the past few weeks. Once current symptoms have been established, the onset of these symptoms is discussed.

The onset starts with the very first symptoms and what was happening when they occurred. Was there some type of accident, repetitive stress, or did it begin spontaneously? The purpose of this is to determine whether the etiology was a stretch injury of the scalene or pectoralis minor muscles resulting in muscle fibrosis and brachial plexus nerve entrapment; or could there have been a direct nerve stretch injury.

3.1. Trauma

Many patients have a history of a traumatic incident, such as a motor vehicle accident or a fall down stairs, on ice or a slippery floor [2]. In the absence of history of an injury, patients should be asked about their occupation, exercise habits, and sports participation, looking for a cause of repetitive stress injury (RSI). RSI occurs in many forms. Working on assembly lines or keyboards are well recognized causes of RSI.

Sports involving a throwing or lifting motion can also produce RSI. However, this RSI causes not only NTOS but is a major cause of NPMS. Because the pectoralis minor muscle attaches to the coracoid process of the scapula, repetitive arm and shoulder movements are the usual etiology of NPMS. This is particularly true in teenagers and young adults who participate in competitive sports. Sports that have been seen to cause NPMS include swimming, baseball (especially pitchers), volleyball, weightlifting, and other activities that have in common scapular retraction stretching the pectoralis minor muscle (PMM) [3].

The history should include whether or not, prior to the onset of the present illness, previous accidents or similar symptoms had occurred. This includes previous trauma or previous surgery for similar symptoms.

3.2. Nerve Injury

The time symptoms develop following an accident is important to document. Paresthesia and/or weakness that occurs immediately after an injury can be due to spinal cord shock or to stretch injuries of nerves of the brachial plexus. If the nerve symptoms disappear in the first few days, spinal shock was the most likely diagnosis. If the symptoms persist, direct nerve injury is likely. In contrast to nerve injury, torn muscles producing nerve compression are the usual cause of paresthesia that develops a few days to many months after the accident and usually progresses over time.

3.3. Spontaneous

A minority of patients have no history of trauma or a specific incident that heralded the onset of symptoms. In such patients, a cervical rib or anomalous first rib can be the etiology. While the majority of patients with rib abnormalities remain asymptomatic throughout their lives, a few of such patients will develop symptoms spontaneously. This is easily detected with a plain cervical spine or chest X-ray.

Once the order of onset of symptoms has been established, the progression or regression of symptoms is determined. This may be related to the treatment provided to date. When recommending therapy to a patient, it is important to know previous treatment and its results. If a patient has already received physical therapy (PT), the specific modalities should be included as some modalities of PT are more helpful than others for NTOS and NPMS.

4. Symptoms

Pain, numbness and/or tingling, and weakness are the common symptoms.

4.1. Pain

The locations of pain are more helpful in the diagnosis than a patient's description of the quality of the pain. Whether the pain is described as "muscular" or "nerve" pain may occasionally help, but, seldom matters. Neck pain and occipital headaches are common in NTOS. Pain or tenderness in the axilla and the anterior chest wall just below the clavicle, strongly suggest NPMS. Pain in the shoulder, upper arm, and forearm is frequent in both of these conditions.

4.2. Paresthesia

Paresthesia is present in over 90% of NTOS and NPMS patients. It usually involves all five fingers, but commonly is worse in the ulnar nerve distribution involving the 4th and 5th fingers.

4.3. Weakness

Weakness is frequently seen, but not as often as pain and paresthesia. Signs of weakness are dropping things and poor grip.

The symptoms in patients with NPMS Alone compared to patients with combined NPMS and NTOS are presented in Table 1. NPMS Alone patients had significantly fewer occipital headaches and pain in the neck, supraclavicular area, and shoulder. When they did have occipital headaches and neck pain, they were usually mild. This was the main difference between the two groups. Weakness occurred less often in the NPMS Alone patients. Significantly more NTOS Alone patients were still working (Table 1) [3].

Table 1. Symptoms of pectoralis minor (PM) alone and with neurogenic thoracic outlet syndrome (NTOS).

	PM Alone	**PM + TOS**	*p* **Value**
Number patients	39	37	
Number operations	52 (N = 52)	48 (N = 52)	
Pain	(No)	(No)	
Occipital Headache	31% (16)	81%(39)	<0.001 *
Neck	50% (26)	96% (46)	<0.001 *
Supraclavicular area	44% (23)	79% (38)	0.004 *
Trapezius	87% (45)	96% (46)	0.163
Pec Minor (Ant. Chest)	69% (36)	92% (44)	0.059
Axilla	52% (27/50)	78% (29/37)	0.024 *
Shoulder	69% (36)	90% (43)	<0.001 *
Arm	71% (37)	88% (42)	0.053
Weakness	58% (30)	88% (42)	0.002 *
Paresthesia	88% (46)	98% (47)	0.114
All 5 fingers	54% (28)	48% (23)	0.699
4th and 5th	29% (15)	42% (20)	0.67
1st–3rd	6% (3)	8% (4)	0.71
None	12% (6)	2% (1)	0.11
Still working	85% (33/39)	57% (21/37)	0.011 *

* ≤0.05, statistically significant difference.

5. Physical Examination

5.1. Tenderness and Tinel's Sign

Physical examination includes investigation for brachial plexus compression at the scalene triangle and under the pectoralis minor muscle. Additionally, evidence is sought for nerve compression at the elbow, forearm, and wrist. These signs include both tenderness and Tinel's sign in each location (Tables 2 and 3).

Table 2. Areas of tenderness.

Signs of Nerve Compression Are the Following:
Tenderness over: 1. Anterior scalene muscle (ASM) and brachial plexus (BP) just above the clavicle   2. Pectoralis minor muscle (PMM) located about one inch below the lateral portion of the clavicle   3. Axilla (associated with pectoralis minor compression)   4. Medial epicondyle over the ulnar nerve (cuboid tunnel)   5. Pronator tunnel   6. Radial tunnel   7. Carpal tunnel   8. Cervical and thoracic spine
Signs of inflammation are tenderness over:
1. Biceps and rotator cuff tendons   2. Trapezius and rhomboid muscles

Table 3. Tinel's sign.

Tinel's Sign is Tested in the Following Areas:
1. Supraclavicular area over the brachial plexus   2. Elbow over the ulnar nerve   3. Pronator tunnel (median nerve)   4. Radial Tunnel (radial nerve)   5. Carpal Tunnel, where Phelan's sign is also tested   6. Guyen's canal (ulnar nerve at wrist)

5.2. Provocative Maneuvers

In addition to palpating for tenderness and checking for positive Tinel's and Phelan's sign, four maneuvers are specific for identifying brachial plexus compression. These are labeled provocative maneuvers and include [4].

5.2.1. Neck Rotation

This is performed by rotating the chin as far as possible towards one shoulder. (Figure 3) Normally, this elicits no symptoms. In NTOS patients, this causes symptoms of pain and/or paresthesia on the opposite (contralateral) side. Symptoms elicited on the same (ipsilateral) side suggest cervical spine disease. This is performed in each direction (to the right, then the left).

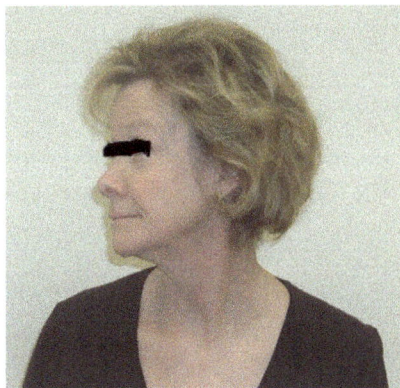

Figure 3. Neck rotation, chin toward shoulder.

5.2.2. Head Tilt

Tilting the head by dropping the ear toward the shoulder normally elicits no symptoms. In NTOS patients, this causes symptoms of pain and paresthesia in the opposite extremity. Symptoms elicited in the same extremity suggest cervical spine disease. Patients with NPMS usually have minimal or no response to neck rotation and head tilt. This maneuver is performed in each direction (Figure 4).

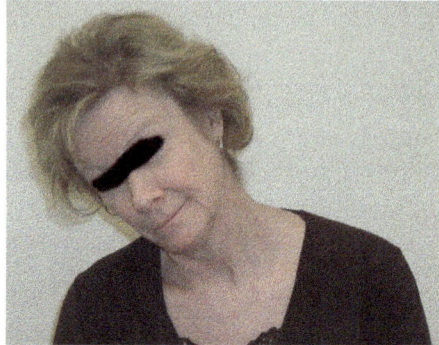

Figure 4. Head tilt, ear to shoulder.

5.2.3. Upper Limb Tension Test (ULTT)

This test is performed by executing three steps: First, the elbows are extended and the arms elevated to 90° parallel to the floor (Figure 5). The second position is dorsiflexion of the wrists. The third position is tilting the head, ear to shoulder, first to the right and then to the left. Normally, no symptoms are elicited. When there is brachial plexus compression, this maneuver brings on the patient's symptoms of pain and paresthesia within a few seconds. The earlier the response, the stronger is the degree of compression; that is, a positive response in position 1 means a stronger degree of compression than just a positive response in position 3 with no responses in positions 1 and 2. This test is comparable to straight leg raising in the lower extremity. It was first described by Elvey and has been modified [5].

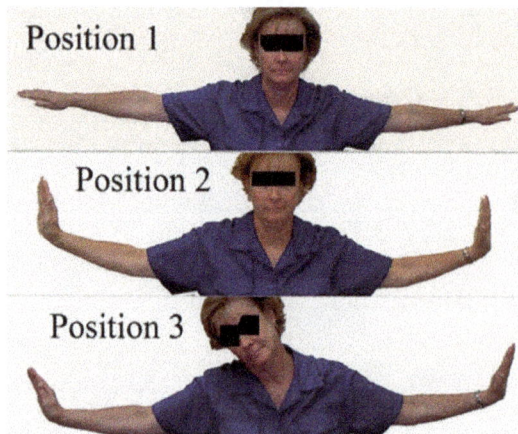

Figure 5. Upper Limb Tension Test (ULTT).

5.2.4. 90° ABD or EAST (Elevated Arm Stress Test)

Abducting the arms to 90° in external rotation (Figure 6). This is also referred to as the Elevated Arm Stress Test or the Roos test. Opening and closing fingers is not necessary. It is the elevation and compression of the neurovascular bundle that is being tested. Finger exercise is indicated only for arterial TOS, when checking for claudication. A positive response is the onset of pain or paresthesia within 60 s. In moderate to severe compression, symptoms often appear within 5 to 30 s.

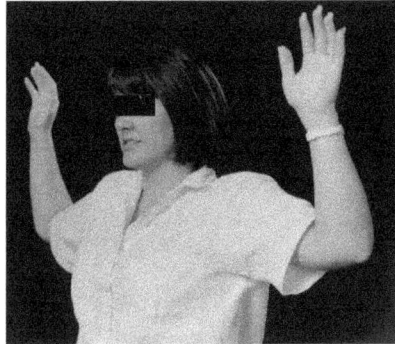

Figure 6. 90° Abduction in External Rotation (90° AER).

6. Numbness

Physical examination includes checking for reduced sensation to light touch in the fingers, comparing one hand to the other. While this can be done with cotton, it can also be done by using the index fingers of the examiners hands lightly touching the bilateral finger tips of the patients hands simultaneously. Each of the five fingers is tested separately. A positive finding is demonstrating reduced sensation to light touch in one or more fingers of one hand compared to the other. The finding of decreased sensation may be present in only some fingers, such as the fourth and fifth fingers.

Findings on physical examination in NPMS Alone patients compared to combined NPMS and NTOS patients are presented in Table 4. While there was no significant difference between NPMS Alone and combined NPMS and NTOS patients in pectoralis minor tenderness, NPMS Alone patients had significantly fewer positive physical findings in all other areas (Table 4) [3].

Table 4. Physical exam–incidence of positive responses.

	PM Alone	PM + TOS	*p* Value
Number patients	39	37	
Number operations	52 (*N* = 52)	48 (*N* = 52)	
Pain	(No)	(No)	
Pec Minor tenderness	92% (48)	100% (48)	0.119
Trapezius tenderness	56% (29)	88% (42)	
Axilla tenderness	71% (32/44)	95% (38/40)	0.008
90° AER	82% (40/50)	100% (45/46)	0.008
ULTT of Elvey	79% (40)	92% (46)	0.008
Scalene tenderness	48% (24)	86% (43)	<0.001
Biceps tenderness	54% (28)	88% (44)	<0.001
Neck rotation	40% (22/51)	80% (41)	<0.001
Head tilt	49% (24/51)	76% (39)	<0.001
Decr. Sensation to Touch	31% (16/51)	48% (23)	<0.001

7. Diagnostic Tests

7.1. Muscle Blocks

Muscle blocks must be distinguished from brachial plexus blocks. A plexus block makes the arm pain free, but also renders it numb and weak. The muscle block relaxes the muscle so it no longer compresses the nerves. After each the muscle block, the physical examination, including the provocative maneuvers, is repeated and the degree of reduction in pain, tenderness, numbness, tingling and weakness. Is recorded.

7.2. Scalene and Pectoralis Minor Muscle Blocks

Injection of 1% Lidocaine into the PMM and ASM is a very useful test to confirm a diagnosis of NTOS and NPMS. These two conditions can exist alone or together. Since becoming aware of NPMS, it has been found that coexistence occurs in at least 75% of the patients seen for NTOS. Therefore, it is important during the physical examination to check for tenderness in both the anterior scalene muscle (ASM) and pectoralis minor muscle (PMM) areas.

The indication to perform a muscle block is a history of pain and elicitation of tenderness over the ASM and/or PMM. When there are positive symptoms and signs in both areas, a block of each muscle is performed during the same examination. The blocks are performed separately; the pectoralis minor block being done first, followed by a repeat physical examination. If all symptoms and signs are gone, the scalene block is not performed. If some symptoms or signs persist, a scalene block is performed and the physical exam repeated again.

7.3. Technique of Muscle Block

The block can be performed with the patient recumbent or sitting. Ultrasound can be used to locate the muscle. In the absence of ultrasound, and with experience, the block can also be performed successfully using standard landmarks. The pectoralis minor landmark is 4–6 cm below the clavicle and over the most tender spot of the PMM; for the scalene, the landmark is through the most tender spot 1–3 cm lateral to the side of trachea and 2 cm above the clavicle. The entry point is always lateral to the carotid pulse and usually through the clavicular head of the sternocleidomastoid muscle. One percent Lidocaine is used for diagnostic blocks because it is short acting. The effect is usually noted within 60 s and usually lasts about 30 min. Should side effects occur from the block, they are gone in a short time.

Pectoralis minor muscle block is performed by injecting 4 mL of 1% Lidocaine through a 5 mL syringe with a 1.5 inch needle. The needle is directed upwards, at a 45° angle, to avoid entering the pleura. The needle entrance is located at the most tender spot 4–5 cm below the clavicle in the region of the PMM. The Lidocaine is injected over an area 1–2 cm deep, and 2 cm wide, by injecting 0.3 to 0.5 mL at a time and moving the needle after each small injection to cover the area. The syringe is aspirated each time the needle is moved to prevent injecting into a blood vessel. If blood is aspirated, the needle is withdrawn a few mm and repositioned in a slightly different direction to avoid the blood vessel. A successful block is indicated by loss of tenderness in the area. If tenderness persists, the procedure can be repeated, aiming the needle in a slightly different direction. Following a successful block, the physical examination is repeated and results recorded. Side effects of the block include increased paresthesia and weakness from Lidocaine spreading to portions of the plexus. These usually wear off in 5–10 min.

The scalene muscle block is performed in similar fashion. Again, aiming the needle cephalad at a 45 degree angle is done to avoid a pneumothorax [1]. Important: where the patient's clavicle projects to make it difficult to achieve a 45 degree angle, the needle is bent to keep the direction cephalad enough to avoid a high lying pleura. When a good block is confirmed by loss of tenderness in the area, the physical examination is repeated once again. Side effects of the scalene block include temporary hoarseness from Lidocaine spreading to a laryngeal nerve or Horner's syndrome due to spread to the sympathetic chain. The authors have not experienced diaphragmatic paralysis.

8. Electrodiagnostic Studies

8.1. Electromyography (EMG)

Until the 1990s, EMG studies were described as normal in most NTOS and NPMS patients. In 1993, measurement of the medial antebrachial sensory cutaneous nerve was introduced [6,7]. Over the next 15 years, further refinement of this technique and normal ranges were developed. This test has proved positive in the large majority of patients operated upon for NTOS and NPMS [8,9].

8.2. C8 Nerve Root Stimulation

This test, though very helpful, is seldom used because it is more painful than most other nerve measurements. It is performed by direct stimulation of the C8 nerve root just outside the cervical spine in the posterior neck. It measures conduction time between the C8 nerve root and a point selected in the neck or arm [9,10].

8.3. Other Tests

8.3.1. A Few Other Techniques Have Been Tried

These have been helpful in occasional cases but not in the majority of NTOS or NPMS patients. These include MRI of the brachial plexus [11] and neurography [12].

8.3.2. X-rays

A plain X-ray of the neck or chest should always be performed to determine whether there is a cervical rib or anomalous first rib. An apical lung mass is rarely discovered (Pancoast tumor).

8.3.3. Associated and Differential Diagnosis

Several conditions can exist with brachial plexus compression as associated conditions and must also be differentiated from it. These conditions are listed in Table 5.

Table 5. Differential and associated diagnoses.

Cervical Spine Disease
Cervical spine strain
Shoulder pathology
Fractured clavicle
Cuboid Tunnel Syndrome (Ulnar nerve entrapment at elbow)
Pronator Tunnel Syndrome
Radial Tunnel Syndrome
Cervical spine disease
Parsnips-Turner Syndrome
Stretch injury of the brachial plexus
Pancoast Tumor

9. Double Crush Syndrome

It is quite common for a second or even a third area of compression to accompany brachial plexus compression. This has been termed "double crush syndrome" [13] or "Triple Crush".

10. Separating NTOS from Neurogenic Pectoralis Minor Syndrome (NPMS)

NTOS usually includes symptoms of neck pain and occipital headaches. NPMS usually includes symptoms of chest pain below the clavicle and in the axilla. Physical examination for NTOS includes significant tenderness over the scalene muscles and radiating pain with pressure over the brachial plexus above the clavicle, and Tinel's sign over the brachial plexus in the neck. NPMS usually has tenderness over the subclavicular area in the region of the PMM and in the axilla. When physical examination includes positive findings in both areas the two conditions usually co-exist. It should be noted that about 75% of the patients seen for NTOS also have symptoms and physical findings of NPMS.

11. Clinical Diagnosis of NPMS Alone Verses NPMS with NTOS

Patients with NPMS Alone usually have a history of repetitive stress activities, particularly competitive sports involving the upper extremities. These include swimming, throwing, volley ball, and weight lifting. Patients with both NTOS and NPMS have histories of motor vehicle accidents or falls down stairs or on ice. In the combined patients, tenderness is usually worse over the anterior chest wall, axilla, and trapezius with less tenderness in the supraclavicular area.

Patients with NTOS alone are more likely to have no headache or neck pain. If these are present, they are minor symptoms.

Physical examination in NPMS Alone patients usually includes tenderness over the pectoralis minor muscle and axilla with little or no tenderness over the scalenes.

12. Treatment of NTOS

Conservative Treatment. Pectoral minor muscle stretching is the most important technique for treating NPMS. This should be recommended for all patients diagnosed with NPMS. It can be performed in a few different ways. We have found standing in an open doorway, with the hands at shoulder level resting on the door jams, is an effective way of achieving this (Figure 7). Patients are instructed to stretch three times a day, hold each stretch for 15 to 20 s, rest for the same length of time, and do three repeats at each session. We suggest three sessions a day, seven days a week. This should be performed for three months. If patients improve enough to be comfortable, nothing else need be done. If there is no significant improvement in three months, they can be offered a pectoralis minor tenotomy, a simple, minimal risk outpatient procedure.

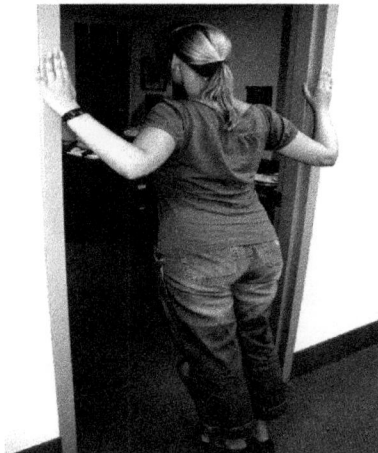

Figure 7. Pectoralis minor stretching. Standing in an open doorway with hands on door jams at shoulder level. Letting the body fall forward stretches the pectoralis minor muscles. The degree of stretching is controlled by the position of the feet either closer to or farther from the threshold line.

13. Surgical Treatment

Currently, results of pectoralis minor stretching are antidotal. A number of patients in whom NPMS was their only diagnosis have achieved good improvement with just one or two months of stretching. These patients continue to do well. The patients in this category had symptoms for less than a year. As part of their treatment, patients stopped the repetitive activity that had elicited their symptoms. Later, they were able to return to that activity, but with less intensity.

Surgical treatment is pectoralis minor tenotomy with partial myomectomy. This can be achieved through either a transaxillary or thoracic approach. Our preference is for the transaxillary approach as it permits wider exposure to completely excise the clavipectoral fascia and any bands or accessory muscles, such as Langer's axillary arch [14], around the axillary neurovascular bundle.

Technique through the axilla begins with a 4–7 cm transverse incision 1–2 cm above the bottom of the axillary hairline, beginning at the anterior axillary fold. The pectoralis major muscle is retracted and the pectoralis minor identified by its attachment to the coracoid process. The origin of pectoralis minor is divided at the coracoid, a 1–2 cm section of the detached muscle end is excised, to prevent reattachment to the brachial plexus. Care is taken to preserve the lateral pectoral nerves to pectoralis major. These nerves traverse through the pectoralis minor and dividing them leads to atrophy of the pectoralis major. Before closure, the clavipectoral fascia and any bands or muscle fibers are excised to leave the neurovascular bundle free of any compressing tissue.

Postoperatively, the remaining body of the pectoralis muscle adheres to the anterior chest wall. To facilitate this adherence, the patient should avoid elevating the arm above shoulder level for 2–3 months after surgery. However, once a day the patient should elevate the arm 180° to avoid a frozen shoulder.

14. Results of Surgical Treatment

Results for pectoralis minor release depend upon whether or not it is associated with NTOS. When NPMS is the only diagnosis, results have been 85% successful. However, when NPMS and NTOS coexist, the success rate for pectoralis minor release alone is closer to 35%. The other 65% may need thoracic outlet decompression at a later date [1,3,15].

15. Oral Informed Consent

Figures 3–6 were of employees of the senior author. Oral informed consent was provided to the author by each subject provided their eyes would be blacked out so identity would be protected.

Author Contributions: Richard J. Sanders annalized the data; Richard J. Sanders and Stephen J. Annest conceived the ideas and wrote the paper.

Conflicts of Interest: The authors declare no conflict of interest.

References

1. Sanders, R.T.; Annest, S.J. Thoracic outlet and pectoralis minor syndromes. *Semin. Vasc. Surg.* **2014**, *27*, 86–117. [CrossRef] [PubMed]
2. Sanders, R.J.; Haug, C.E. *Thoracic Outlet Syndrome: A Common Sequela of Neck Injuries*; Lippincott: Philadelphia, PA, USA, 1991; p. 26.
3. Sanders, R.J.; Rao, N.M. The forgotten pectoralis minor syndrome: 100 operations for pectoralis minor syndrome alone or accompanied by neurogenic thoracic outlet syndrome. *Ann. Vasc. Surg.* **2010**, *24*, 701–708. [CrossRef] [PubMed]
4. Sanders, R.J.; Hammond, S.L. Diagnosis of thoracic outlet syndrome. *J. Vasc. Surg.* **2007**, *46*, 601–604. [CrossRef] [PubMed]
5. Elvey, R.L. The investigation of arm pain. In *Modern Manual Therapy of the Vertebral Column*; Churchill Livingstone: Edinburgh, UK, 1986; pp. 530–535.

6. Nishida, T.; Price, S.J.; Minieka, M.M. Medial antebrachial cutaneous nerve conduction in true neurogenic thoracic outlet syndrome. *Electromyogr. Clin. Neurophysiol.* **1993**, *33*, 255–258.
7. Kothari, M.J.; Macintosh, K.; Heistand, M.; Logigian, E.L. Medial antebrachial cutaneous sensory studies in the evaluation of neurogenic thoracic outlet syndrome. *Muscle Nerve* **1998**, *21*, 647–649. [CrossRef]
8. Seror, P. Medial antebrachial cutaneous nerve conduction study, a new tool to demonstrate mild lower brachial plexus lesions. A report of 16 cases. *Clin. Neurophysiol.* **2004**, *115*, 2316–2322. [CrossRef] [PubMed]
9. Machanic, B.I.; Sanders, R.J. Medial antebrachial cutaneous nerve measurements to diagnose neurogenic thoracic outlet syndrome. *Ann. Vasc. Surg.* **2008**, *22*, 248–254. [CrossRef] [PubMed]
10. Papathanasiou, E.; Zamba, E.; Papacostas, S. Normative values for high voltage electrical stimulation across the brachial plexus. *Electromyogr. Clin. Neurophysiol.* **2002**, *42*, 151–157. [PubMed]
11. Boulanger, X.; Ledoux, J.B.; Brun, A.L.; Beigellman, C. Imaging of the non-traumatic brachial plexus. *Diagn. Interv. Imaging* **2013**, *94*, 945–956. [CrossRef] [PubMed]
12. Filler, A. Magnetic resonance neurography and diffusion tensor imaging: Origins, history, and clinical impact of the first 50,000 cases with an assessment of efficacy and utility in a prospective 5000-patient study group. *Neurosurgery* **2009**, *65*, A29–A43. [CrossRef] [PubMed]
13. Upton, A.R.M.; McComas, A.J. The double crush in nerve-entrapment syndromes. *Lancet* **1973**, *2*, 359–362. [CrossRef]
14. Magee, C.; Jones, C.; MacIntosh, S.; Harkin, D.W. Upper limb deep vein thrombosis due to Langer's axillary arch. *J. Vasc. Surg.* **2012**, *55*, 234–236. [CrossRef] [PubMed]
15. Sanders, R.J.; Annest, S.J.; Goldson, E. Neurogenic thoracic outlet and pectoralis minor syndromes in children. *Vasc. Endovasc. Surg.* **2013**, *47*, 335–341. [CrossRef] [PubMed]

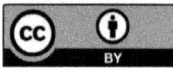

diagnostics

MDPI

Article

Long-Term Functional Outcome of Surgical Treatment for Thoracic Outlet Syndrome

Jesse Peek [1], Cornelis G. Vos [2], Çağdas Ünlü [2], Michiel A. Schreve [2], Rob H. W. van de Mortel [1] and Jean-Paul P. M. de Vries [1,*]

[1] Department of Vascular Surgery, St Antonius Hospital, 3435CM Nieuwegein, The Netherlands;
     j.peek@students.uu.nl (J.P.); r.van.de.mortel@antoniusziekenhuis.nl (R.H.W.v.d.M.)
[2] Department of Vascular Surgery, Medical Center Alkmaar, 1815JD Alkmaar, The Netherlands;
     ncgvos@gmail.com (C.G.V.); cagdas.unlu@nwz.nl (Ç.Ü.); m.schreve@nwz.nl (M.A.S.)
*   Correspondence: j.vries@antoniusziekenhuis.nl; Tel.: +31-(0)883-201-925

Received: 14 December 2017; Accepted: 11 January 2018; Published: 12 January 2018

Abstract: First rib resection for thoracic outlet syndrome (TOS) is clinically successful and safe in most patients. However, long-term functional outcomes are still insufficiently known. Long-term functional outcome was assessed using a validated questionnaire. A multicenter retrospective cohort study including all patients who underwent operations for TOS from January 2005 until December 2016. Clinical records were reviewed and the long-term functional outcome was assessed by the 11-item version of the Disability of the Arm, Shoulder, and Hand (QuickDASH) questionnaire. Sixty-two cases of TOS in 56 patients were analyzed: 36 neurogenic TOS, 13 arterial TOS, 7 venous TOS, and 6 combined TOS. There was no 30-day mortality. One reoperation because of bleeding was performed and five patients developed a pneumothorax. Survey response was 73% (*n* = 41) with a follow-up ranging from 1 to 11 years. Complete relief of symptoms was reported postoperatively in 27 patients (54%), symptoms improved in 90%, and the mean QuickDASH score was 22 (range, 0–86). Long-term functional outcome of surgical treatment of TOS was satisfactory, and surgery was beneficial in 90% of patients, with a low risk of severe morbidity. However, the mean QuickDASH scores remain higher compared with the general population, suggesting some sustained functional impairment despite clinical improvement of symptoms.

Keywords: thoracic outlet syndrome; first rib resection; surgical procedures; operative; patient reported outcome measures

1. Introduction

Thoracic outlet syndrome (TOS) is caused by compression of the neurovascular bundle (brachial plexus, subclavian vein or artery) in the thoracic outlet. TOS can be grouped as neurogenic and vascular, depending on the anatomical structure that is compromised. Neurogenic TOS (NTOS), the most common form (95–99%), is caused by compression of the brachial plexus. Neurological symptoms, such as pain, paresthesia, numbness, Raynaud phenomenon, and/or weakness in arm and shoulder, have been described. Vascular TOS, caused by compression of the subclavian vessels below the clavicle, includes venous TOS (VTOS) and arterial TOS (ATOS) and is relatively uncommon [1,2].

TOS, especially NTOS, is a poorly understood condition, and the diagnosis is highly debatable because there are no objective, well-defined, diagnostic criteria. Furthermore, diagnosing NTOS is a challenging task because of the variability of presenting symptoms and the lack of sensitive and specific diagnostic tests.

Physiotherapy and additional medication (i.e., painkillers, anti-inflammatory medications, or muscle relaxants) are the mainstays of management of NTOS, and together they may improve arm function and reduce symptoms. If conservative treatment fails, surgical treatment may be considered for patients with persisting symptoms [2,3]. Management and presentation are different in the case of vascular involvement, and surgery is preferred in a larger proportion of patients [2,3].

Many publications have appeared in recent decades documenting different surgical approaches and their outcomes. Surgical interventions seem beneficial for most patients, although patient selection is important [4]. Significant improvements in arm function in both the neurogenic and vascular group was observed [4]. However, high-quality studies, including those with large enough sample sizes and using validated outcome measures to describe results of treatment, are lacking. Thus, the main objective of this study was to evaluate the long-term functional outcomes for surgically treated patients with TOS.

2. Materials and Methods

The Medical Ethics Review Boards of St. Antonius Hospital (MEC-U Nieuwegein) and Medical Center Alkmaar (METC Noord-Holland, Alkmaar, The Netherlands) The Netherlands approved the study (6 July 2016, R&D/Z16.061), and informed consent was obtained for all patients.

2.1. Patient Selection

This retrospective, multicenter, medical record review was performed at the departments of vascular surgery of two large vascular referral centers. The study enrolled all patients with unilateral or bilateral first or cervical rib resection for TOS of any type from January 2005 until December 2016. The extracted data included patient characteristics, type of TOS, and the presenting symptoms and signs, including pain, numbness, and loss of strength in arm, neck, or shoulder. Thrombotic signs, medical history, preceding trauma, risk factors, intoxications, and other complaints were also recorded. Information from the diagnostic workup included data of physical examination (e.g., Roos Elevated Arm Stress Test, Adson test, and Allen test) and data from additional radiographic imaging, including phlebographies, arteriographies, duplex ultrasonography with additional provocation testing, computed tomography scans (CT), or magnetic resonance imaging (MRI). Also collected was the type of operation, outcomes of additional therapy (thrombolysis, percutaneous transluminal angioplasty, or vascular reconstruction), and follow-up information.

2.2. Workup and Surgical Intervention

The workup for patients with symptoms indicating TOS depended on the type of TOS. An important part of the work-up for NTOS patients consisted of ruling out other pathology that could cause similar symptoms. This included imaging studies—such as duplex ultrasonography with provocation testing, CT, or MRI—and referral to a neurologist to rule out other neurogenic causes such as radicular compression or peripheral nerve compression. The first step in treatment was always a conservative management, including counseling, physiotherapy and injections with anesthetics, steroids, or Botox. When conservative management failed to improve symptoms, surgery for thoracic outlet decompression was offered.

VTOS patients, usually presenting with venous thrombosis, were treated conservatively (i.e., anticoagulation and compression stocking therapy) or, depending on the severity of the deep venous thrombotic symptoms, by catheter directed thrombolysis, followed by first rib resection if thrombolysis was successful. Depending on residual venous lesions, subsequent endovascular treatment (percutaneous transluminal angioplasty with eventual additional stenting) or venous reconstruction was performed after the first rib resection.

ATOS was only treated surgically in symptomatic patients. This could be disabling claudication not responding to supervised exercise therapy of the arm or critical upper extremity ischemia resulting from subclavian artery obstruction or by peripheral embolization caused by a subclavian artery aneurysm. If needed, catheter-directed thrombolysis was performed first, followed by first rib resection, and in case of residual vascular lesions (stenosis or aneurysm), a reconstruction or endovascular treatment was performed subsequently.

The standard surgical approach in both institutions was a first rib resection through a transaxillary approach, as described by Roos et al. [5]. A wound suction drain was usually sufficient to allow complete expansion of the lung if pleural defects occurred during dissection. A chest tube was inserted in cases of persistent pneumothorax. Postoperative pain was managed using a preoperatively given scalene nerve block and intravenous opioids, and early mobilization and physiotherapy were prescribed. In some cases of VTOS, an infraclavicular approach was preferred for better exposure of the subclavian vein [6]. For ATOS and occasionally for cervical ribs, a supraclavicular approach was preferred [6]. Patients were referred to a physiotherapist postoperatively and received instructions to limit abduction to 90° for the first two weeks. After two weeks, no limitations and active mobilization was prescribed. A routine follow-up visit was planned for all patients six weeks postoperatively.

2.3. Long-Term Outcome

For the assessment of the functional and surgical outcomes, all patients were contacted by telephone and were, after agreement for participation was obtained, asked to complete a validated questionnaire. The 11-item version of the Disabilities of the Arm, Shoulder and Hand (QuickDASH) questionnaire was used to assess the subjective disability of arm and shoulder function [7–9]. The QuickDASH questionnaire is validated and frequently used in functional studies after upper extremity operations [7–9]. A higher score (maximum 100) implies a higher subjective disability of arm and shoulder function. A score of 0 represents optimal function. The questionnaire has two optional modules assessing work and sports, which were only used with patients who worked or were engaged in any sports activities. The questionnaire is available on http://www.dash.iwh.on.ca/about-quickdash.

2.4. Statistical Analysis

All patient information was put into a database created in SPSS 23.0 software (IBM, Armonk, NY, USA) for statistical analysis. Continuous variables are expressed as medians with ranges.

3. Results

3.1. Patient Characteristics

Between January 2005 and December 2016, 56 patients with TOS underwent a first rib resection and 18 also underwent a cervical rib resection. Six patients were treated bilaterally; therefore, the study included a total of 62 surgical procedures. All patients were contacted and asked to complete and return the QuickDASH questionnaire. Follow-up data were available at 30 days for all patients, and all attended the first postoperative visit at four to six weeks. Of the 56 patients, 41 (73%) returned a completely filled-out questionnaire. Reasons for nonresponders included could not be reached by telephone or mail ($n = 6$), refused to complete the questionnaire ($n = 3$), and death from a cause unrelated to the operation or TOS ($n = 2$). Four patients who initially agreed to participate in the study never returned their questionnaires despite several reminders. The interval between the operation and completing the QuickDASH questionnaire was at least one year (range, 1–11 years). Characteristics of the patients who did and did not respond are summarized in Table 1.

Table 1. Patient characteristics.

Characteristics	Responders ($n = 41$)	Non-Responders ($n = 15$)
Male sex	16 (39%)	5 (33%)
Age	43 (17–64)	40 (21–64)
ASA 1/2	41 (100%)	13 (87%)

Table 1. *Cont.*

Characteristics		Responders (*n* = 41)	Non-Responders (*n* = 15)
Smoking		14 (34%)	6 (40%)
Type of TOS	NTOS	26 (63%)	10 (67%)
	VTOS	7 (17%)	0 (0%)
	ATOS	10 (24%)	3 (20%)
	Combined	4 (10%)	2 (13%)
Bilateral TOS		6 (14%)	0 (0%)
Cervical rib		13 (28%)	5 (33%)
Athlete		1 (2%)	0 (0%)

Values are *n* (%) or median (range). Abbreviations: TOS—thoracic outlet syndrome; NTOS—neurogenic thoracic outlet syndrome; VTOS—venous thoracic outlet syndrome; ATOS—arterial thoracic outlet syndrome.

3.2. Surgical Procedure and Complications

Transaxillary first rib resections were performed in 51 of the 62 surgical procedures. A supraclavicular approach was performed in nine cases to remove cervical ribs (*n* = 6) or reconstruct the subclavian artery (ATOS; *n* = 3). Two patients underwent an infraclavicular approach and subclavian vein reconstruction because of VTOS. In the remaining ATOS (*n* = 10) and VTOS (*n* = 7) patients, an additional percutaneous transluminal angioplasty with stent placement was performed after resection of the first rib.

Pleural damage during the operation in five patients resulted in a pneumothorax that required chest tube drainage. One patient underwent a reoperation because of postoperative bleeding. No wound infections or other infectious complications occurred, and no transient or permanent motor nerve injury was observed. The 30-day mortality rate was 0.

3.3. Functional Outcome and QuickDASH

At long-term follow-up (i.e., ≥1 year), 27 patients (54%) reported complete relief of symptoms. The remaining patients reported minor remaining paresthesia in the ipsilateral arm (*n* = 2), some persisting pain in the ipsilateral arm or shoulder (*n* = 14), or a recurrence of the preoperative complaints (*n* = 8). After 56 of the 62 interventions (90%), patients reported an improvement of their symptoms during the last visit at the outpatient clinic.

The median QuickDASH score for the 41 responders was 22 (range, 0–86). The median score was 18 (range, 0–63) for the work module (*n* = 28) and was 23 (range, 0–100) for the sports module (*n* = 27).

4. Discussion

The present study evaluated the long-term functional outcome of surgically treated patients with TOS. A complete resolution of symptoms was reported by 54% of the patients, and clinical improvement was obtained in 90% of patients. Median scores at a follow-up of at least one year postoperatively were 22 for the QuickDASH, 18 for the optional work module, and 22 for the optional sports module. These scores were all slightly higher compared with the values found in the general population in the United States, where these score were 10, 9, and 10, respectively [10]. Apparently, TOS patients continue to experience more functional impairment compared with the general population, despite surgical treatment. Although most patients reported an improvement of symptoms, only 39% had a mean QuickDASH score of 10 or lower. This suggests that even though preoperative symptoms improve, some functional impairment can remain and might be partly caused by the surgical procedure. However, the data of the present study are not sufficient to prove this hypothesis.

Several other studies have reported DASH scores after surgical treatment for TOS ranging from 3.5 to 36 [11–16]. Functional outcome as reported by DASH scores is better in athletes [11] and in vascular forms of TOS [14,16]. The explanation for the differences in the outcome between vascular forms of TOS and NTOS is that a substantial number of patients with VTOS or ATOS also undergo revascularization procedures. There is also some evidence indicating that early treatment ($\leq$3 months) might result in better functional outcome than delayed (>6 months) treatment [12,13]. A hypothesis to explain this benefit of early treatment is the prevention of further nerve degeneration and muscle wasting caused by the compression at the thoracic outlet [13]. A meta-analysis by Peek et al. [4] found a mean improvement in the DASH score of 28.3 points after surgical treatment for TOS. Furthermore, an overall clinical success of $\geq$90% was found for vascular forms of TOS and was 60–80% for the NTOS patients [4].

The diagnosis of NTOS especially remains a challenge for many physicians and might be an important explanation for the relatively disappointing outcomes of surgical treatment of NTOS compared with ATOS and VTOS. Although there are several diagnostic provocation tests, such as the elevation arm stress test and the Adson test, or a trial scalene block, these tests depend on (subjective) patient-reported symptoms. More objective parameters for the diagnosis of NTOS are required. MRI or CT angiography might be used to identify evidence for compression at the thoracic outlet.

Patient selection could also be improved by obtaining disease-specific validated questionnaires that use discriminating signs and symptoms. Balderman et al. [17] recently described clinical diagnostic criteria that can help to diagnose NTOS. In a cohort of 183 patients referred with NTOS, the most frequently positive pretreatment criteria were neck or upper extremity pain (99%), upper extremity or hand paresthesia (94%), symptom exacerbation by arm elevation (97%), localized supraclavicular or subcoracoid tenderness to palpation (96%), and a positive three-minute elevated arm stress test (94%). Further research is needed to confirm these findings and to correlate these pretreatment criteria with clinical outcome [17].

Another future diagnostic approach could include sensitive nerve conduction studies or imaging studies of the thoracic outlet in different provocative positions of the extremities.

There are several limitations that influence the conclusions that can be drawn from this study. The retrospective nature implies a risk of selection bias, although all consecutively operated-on patients were included. The sample size of 62 patients is reasonable compared with previous studies, although this sample was acquired over a period of approximately 11 years (2005–2016). As a result of the interval between surgery and patients completing the questionnaires, the influence of other factors or events on functional performance cannot be ruled out. Unfortunately, our study did not include data on conservatively managed patients, and therefore, a comparison between conservative and surgical treatment could not be made. Because of the retrospective design, we had no data on baseline QuickDASH scores and could not compare preoperative and postoperative functional outcomes. Finally, the heterogeneity within the study cohort (types of TOS, surgical approach) and the sample size precluded reliable regression analysis to identify factors predictive for a functional outcome.

5. Conclusions

In conclusion, long-term functional outcome of surgical treatment in TOS patients is satisfactory, and surgery is beneficial in most patients. However, the mean QuickDASH scores remain higher compared with the general population, suggesting some functional impairment remains despite clinical improvement of symptoms.

Acknowledgments: The authors received no financial support for the research, authorship, and/or publication of this article.

Author Contributions: Jesse Peek data collection, data analysis, draft of the manuscript; Cornelis G. Vos data analysis and interpretation, revision of the manuscript; Çağdas Ünlü study design, data analysis and interpretation, revision of the manuscript; Michiel A. Schreve data interpretation, revision of the manuscript; Rob H. W. van de Mortel data interpretation, revision of the manuscript; Jean-Paul P. M. de Vries study design, data analysis and interpretation, revision of the manuscript; All authors read and approved the final manuscript.

Conflicts of Interest: The authors declare no conflict of interest.

References

1. Fugate, M.W.; Rotellini-Coltvet, L.; Freischlag, J.A. Current management of thoracic outlet syndrome. *Curr. Treat. Opt. Cardiovasc. Med.* **2009**, *11*, 176–183. [CrossRef]
2. Sanders, R.J.; Hammond, S.L.; Rao, N.M. Diagnosis of thoracic outlet syndrome. *J. Vasc. Surg.* **2007**, *46*, 601–604. [CrossRef] [PubMed]
3. Desai, Y.; Robbs, J.V. Arterial complications of the thoracic outlet syndrome. *Eur. J. Vasc. Endovasc. Surg.* **1995**, *10*, 362–365. [CrossRef]
4. Peek, J.; Vos, C.G.; Unlu, C.; van de Pavoordt, H.D.; van den Akker, P.J.; de Vries, J.P. Outcome of Surgical Treatment for Thoracic Outlet Syndrome: Systematic Review and Meta-Analysis. *Ann. Vasc. Surg.* **2017**, *40*, 303–326. [CrossRef] [PubMed]
5. Roos, D.B. Transaxillary approach for first rib resection to relieve thoracic outlet syndrome. *Ann. Surg.* **1966**, *163*, 354–358. [CrossRef] [PubMed]
6. Vos, C.G.; Ünlü, C.; Voûte, M.T.; Van de Mortel, R.H.W.; De Vries, J.P.P.M. Thoracic outlet syndrome: First rib resection. In *Shanghai Chest*; AME Books Publishing: Hongkong, China, 2017; Volume 1, p. 3.
7. Hudak, P.; Amadio, P.C.; Bombardier, C.; Upper Extremity Collaborative Group. Development of an upper extremity outcome measure: The DASH (Disabilities of the Arm, Shoulder, and Hand). *Am. J. Ind. Med.* **1996**, *29*, 602–608. [CrossRef]
8. Beaton, D.E.; Katz, J.N.; Fossel, A.H.; Wright, J.G.; Tarasuk, V.; Bombardier, C. Measuring the whole or the parts? Validity, reliability & responsiveness of the disabilities of the arm, shoulder, and hand outcome measure in diferent regions of the upper extremity. *J. Hand Ther.* **2001**, *14*, 128–146. [PubMed]
9. Beaton, D.E.; Wright, J.G.; Katz, J.N.; Upper Extremity Collaborative Group. Development of the QuickDASH: Comparison of three item-reduction approaches. *J. Bone Jt. Surg. Am.* **2005**, *87A*, 1038–1046.
10. Hunsaker, F.G.; Cioffi, D.A.; Amadio, P.C.; Wright, J.G.; Caughlin, B. The American academy of orthopaedic surgeons outcomes instruments: Normative values from the general population. *J Bone Jt. Surg. Am.* **2002**, *84-A*, 208–215. [CrossRef]
11. Chandra, V.; Little, C.; Lee, J.T. Thoracic outlet syndrome in high-performance athletes. *J. Vasc. Surg.* **2014**, *60*, 1012–1017. [CrossRef] [PubMed]
12. Elixène, J.B.; Sadaghianloo, N.; Mousnier, A.; Brizzi, S.; Declemy, S.; Hassen-Khodja, R. Long-term functional outcomes and subclavian vein patency in patients undergoing thoracic outlet surgery for Paget-Schroetter Syndrome. *J. Cardiovasc. Surg.* **2017**, *58*, 451–457.
13. Al-Hashel, J.Y.; El Shorbgy, A.A.; Ahmed, S.F.; Elshereef, R.R. Early versus Late Surgical Treatment for Neurogenic Thoracic Outlet Syndrome. *ISRN Neurol.* **2013**, *2013*, 673020. [CrossRef] [PubMed]
14. Glynn, R.W.; Tawfick, W.; Elsafty, Z.; Hynes, N.; Sultan, S. Supraclavicular scalenectomy for thoracic outlet syndrome—Functional outcomes assessed using the DASH scoring system. *Vasc. Endovasc. Surg.* **2012**, *46*, 157–162. [CrossRef] [PubMed]
15. Chandra, V.; Olcott, C., 4th; Lee, J.T. Early results of a highly selective algorithm for surgery on patients with neurogenic thoracic outlet syndrome. *J. Vasc. Surg.* **2011**, *54*, 1698–1705. [CrossRef] [PubMed]
16. Cordobes-Gual, J.; Lozano-Vilardell, P.; Torreguitart-Mirada, N.; Lara-Hernandez, R.; Riera-Vazquez, R.; Julia-Montoya, J. Prospective study of the functional recovery after surgery for thoracic outlet syndrome. *Eur. J. Vasc. Endovasc. Surg.* **2008**, *35*, 79–83. [CrossRef] [PubMed]
17. Balderman, J.; Holzem, K.; Field, B.J.; Bottros, M.M.; Abuirqeba, A.A.; Vemuri, C.; Thompson, R.W. Associations between clinical diagnostic criteria and pretreatment patient-reported outcomes measures in a prospective observational cohort of patients with neurogenic thoracic outlet syndrome. *J. Vasc. Surg.* **2017**, *66*, 533–544. [CrossRef] [PubMed]

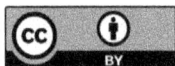

diagnostics

MDPI

Article

A Patient-Centered Approach to Guide Follow-Up and Adjunctive Testing and Treatment after First Rib Resection for Venous Thoracic Outlet Syndrome Is Safe and Effective

Colin P. Ryan [1], Nicolas J. Mouawad [2], Patrick S. Vaccaro [1] and Michael R. Go [1,*]

[1] Division of Vascular Diseases and Surgery, The Ohio State University College of Medicine, Columbus, OH 43210, USA; cryan7209@gmail.com (C.P.R.); patrick.vaccaro@osumc.edu (P.S.V.)

[2] McClaren Bay Heart and Vascular, McClaren Regional Medical Center, Flint, MI 48532, USA; nicolas.mouawad@osumc.edu

* Correspondence: Michael.go@osumc.edu; Tel.: +1-614-293-8536

Received: 2 January 2018; Accepted: 19 January 2018; Published: 23 January 2018

Abstract: Controversies in the treatment of venous thoracic outlet syndrome (VTOS) have been discussed for decades, but still persist. Calls for more objective reporting standards have pushed practice towards comprehensive venous evaluations and interventions after first rib resection (FRR) for all patients. In our practice, we have relied on patient-centered, patient-reported outcomes to guide adjunctive treatment and measure success. Thus, we sought to investigate the use of thrombolysis versus anticoagulation alone, timing of FRR following thrombolysis, post-FRR venous intervention, and FRR for McCleery syndrome (MCS) and their impact on patient symptoms and return to function. All patients undergoing FRR for VTOS at our institution from 4 April 2000 through 31 December 2013 were reviewed. Demographics, symptoms, diagnostic and treatment details, and outcomes were collected. Per "Reporting Standards of the Society for Vascular Surgery for Thoracic Outlet Syndrome", symptoms were described as swelling/discoloration/heaviness, collaterals, concomitant neurogenic symptoms, and functional impairment. Patient-reported response to treatment was defined as complete (no residual symptoms and return to function), partial (any residual symptoms present but no functional impairment), temporary (initial improvement but subsequent recurrence of any symptoms or functional impairment), or none (persistent symptoms or functional impairment). Sixty FRR were performed on 59 patients. 54.2% were female with a mean age of 34.3 years. Swelling/discoloration/heaviness was present in all but one patient, deep vein thrombosis in 80%, and visible collaterals in 41.7%. Four patients had pulmonary embolus while 65% had concomitant neurogenic symptoms. In addition, 74.6% of patients were anticoagulated and 44.1% also underwent thrombolysis prior to FRR. Complete or partial response occurred in 93.4%. Of the four patients with temporary or no response, further diagnostics revealed residual venous disease in two and occult alternative diagnoses in two. Use of thrombolysis was not related to FRR outcomes ($p = 0.600$). Performance of FRR less than or greater than six weeks after the initiation of anticoagulation or treatment with thrombolysis was not related to FRR outcomes ($p = 1$). Whether patients had DVT or MCS was not related to FRR outcomes ($p = 1$). No patient had recurrent DVT. From a patient-centered, patient-reported standpoint, VTOS is equally effectively treated with FRR regardless of preoperative thrombolysis or timing of surgery after thrombolysis. A conservative approach to venous interrogation and intervention after FRR is safe and effective for symptom control and return to function. Additionally, patients with MCS are effectively treated with FRR.

Keywords: venous thoracic outlet syndrome; thoracic outlet syndrome; first rib resection; thoracic outlet decompression; thrombolysis; Paget-Schroetter syndrome; McCleery syndrome; deep venous thrombosis

1. Introduction

Controversies in the treatment of venous thoracic outlet syndrome (VTOS) include the use of preoperative thrombolysis, timing of first rib resection (FRR) after presentation, surgical approach, and the role of post-FRR venous intervention. The lack of true comparative analysis data in thoracic outlet syndrome in general, and VTOS in particular, has resulted in calls for objective reporting criteria and an emphasis on diagnostics to measure treatment success [1–3].

While this clearly fills an important and well-recognized gap in the VTOS literature, in our practice we have historically focused on patient-centered, patient-reported measures of treatment success, and thus do not pursue duplex or venography after FRR, and do not treat incidentally identified lesions, unless the patient has significant residual symptoms or functional impairment. In this setting, our patient population is suited to address some of the existing controversies in the treatment of VTOS, especially as they relate to patient-reported outcomes and conservative management of residual venous disease after FRR.

Thus, in a practice emphasizing patient-reported outcomes over venous patency, we sought to describe the effect of pre-operative thrombolysis, timing of FRR, and a conservative approach to post-operative vein management on the results of treatment of VTOS. Additionally, we investigated the role of FRR in the treatment of symptoms and functional impairment from McCleery syndrome (MCS).

2. Materials and Methods

This study was approved by the Ohio State University Institutional Review Board (Protocol 2013H0067 approved 2/22/13 with ongoing approval). A retrospective review analyzing all patients undergoing FRR for VTOS from 4 April 2000 through 31 December 2013 at our institution was performed. VTOS was defined according to the "Reporting Standards of the Society for Vascular Surgery for Thoracic Outlet Syndrome" as a presence of consistent history, consistent examination, and imaging demonstrating DVT or venous abnormality at the thoracic outlet, with the exception that asymptomatic incidentally found venous compression without DVT was not treated [3]. No patients had concomitant arterial TOS, but some did have neurogenic symptoms.

Also per "Reporting Standards of the Society for Vascular Surgery for Thoracic Outlet Syndrome", symptoms were described as swelling/discoloration/heaviness, collaterals, concomitant neurogenic symptoms, and functional impairment; this data was collected for all patients in our practice, including those treated prior to the publication of the reporting standards.

Patients presenting with VTOS and DVT all were anticoagulated for a total of three months from presentation. Patients underwent additional pre-operative thrombolysis based on the judgment of the treating surgeon. If thrombolysis occurred, it was performed using ultrasound-accelerated thrombolysis (EKOS Corporation, Bothell, WA, USA) while infusing 1 mg/h tPA for 12–24 h. Venoplasty for residual stenosis after thrombolysis was performed using low pressure, smaller diameter balloons only as a temporizing measure, and stents were avoided. The decision of when to perform FRR after anticoagulation and thrombolysis was made by the treating surgeon, and all FRR were performed via the transaxillary approach with anterior scalenotomy and external venolysis but without venous reconstruction.

Response to treatment included outcomes defined in "Reporting Standards of the Society for Vascular Surgery for Thoracic Outlet Syndrome", including overall subjective status, return to function, objective examination, and—most importantly—patient-reported symptoms. Response was further defined as complete (no residual symptoms and return to function), partial (any residual symptoms present but no functional impairment), temporary (initial improvement but subsequent recurrence of any symptoms or functional impairment), or none (persistent symptoms or functional impairment), similar to the methodology of Derkash et al. and subsequently utilized by Degeorges et al. [4,5]. Outcomes were further categorized as favorable or unfavorable, as done by Orlando et al. [6]. Patients were considered to have complete response only if absolutely no swelling, discoloration, heaviness, collaterals, or any upper extremity symptoms of any kind were reported or identified on exam.

Follow-up was heavily influenced by patient-reported symptoms and functional outcomes rather than anatomic or patency measures. All patients returned at one month for a history and examination. Those with no residual symptoms had no further follow-up or assessments arranged, but were told to return if any symptoms recurred. In any patient with residual symptoms or functional limitation, further venous interrogation and intervention were undertaken.

Data were stored in a password-protected database on a secured computer. Deidentified data were imported to SPSS (Version 22, IBM Corporation, Armonk, NY, USA) for statistical analysis. Summaries of the entire cohort were created using medians and ranges for continuous measures and frequencies and percentages for categorical measures. Chi-squared analysis of outcomes measures for variables with expected counts greater than five was performed. Fisher exact testing was utilized for variables with expected counts less than five.

3. Results

Sixty FRR in 59 patients were performed for VTOS. DVT was diagnosed in 48 patients (80%), while MCS was diagnosed in 12 (20%).

Table 1 shows summaries of the demographic and presenting features of the VTOS cohort. Favorable outcome indicates complete or partial response. Patients presenting with venous distention were more likely to have an unfavorable outcome.

Table 1. Association of patient presentation variables with surgical outcomes.

Factor	Number (%)	% Favorable Outcome	p-Value
Gender			
Male	28 (45.8%)	92.8%	1
Female	32 (54.2%)	93.8%	1
Smoking Status			
Nonsmoker	45 (70.3%)	95.6%	-
Past/Current Smoker	15 (29.7%)	86.7%	0.258
Occupation			
Unemployed/Disabled/Retired	18 (30.5%)	88.8%	0.572
Student/Sedentary Laborer	14 (23.3%)	92.4%	1
Student Athlete	17 (28.3%)	91.4%	1
Overhead/Physical Laborer	10 (16.7%)	90%	1
Presentation			
Upper Extremity Swelling	59 (98.3%)	-	1
Venous Distension	25 (41.7%)	84.0%	0.026
Deep Venous Thrombosis	48 (80%)	94.0%	0.528
Pulmonary Embolus	4 (6.7%)	100%	1
Neurologic Symptoms	39 (65%)	92.3%	1
Family Clotting History	9 (15%)	100%	1

Twenty-seven patients were female with a mean age of 34.3 years. Eight patients (13.6%) had a family history of coagulopathy and one patient had a parent with VTOS. Thirty-one percent of patients were unemployed or disabled, 28.8% were athletes, 16.9% were sedentary workers, and 16.9% were repetitive overhead workers.

Swelling was present in 98.3% (97.9% of patients with DVT, 100% of patients with MCS). Venous distention was present in 41.7% (35.4% of patients with DVT, 58.3% of patients with MCS). Four patients had pulmonary embolus at presentation. Sixty-five percent had concurrent upper extremity neurologic symptoms.

Regarding treatment, 78% of patients were anticoagulated (95.8% of patients with DVT, 0% of patients with MCS). In addition, 54.1% of patients with DVT underwent thrombolysis prior to FRR. Overall, complete response was achieved in 71.7% of patients, partial response was achieved in 21.7%, and temporary or no response each occurred in 3.3% (Figure 1).

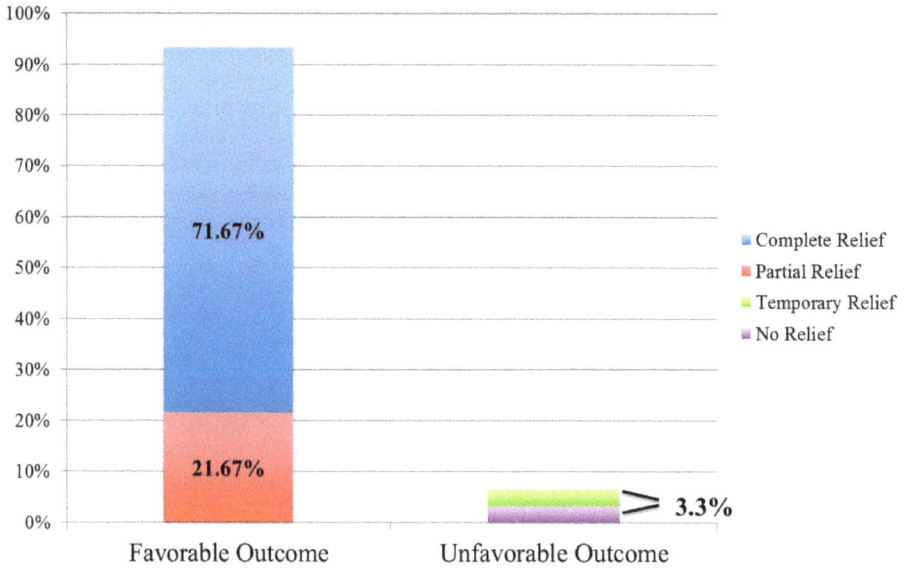

Figure 1. Response following first rib resection (FRR).

Performance of preoperative thrombolysis was not related to FRR outcomes ($p = 0.620$) as demonstrated in Figure 2.

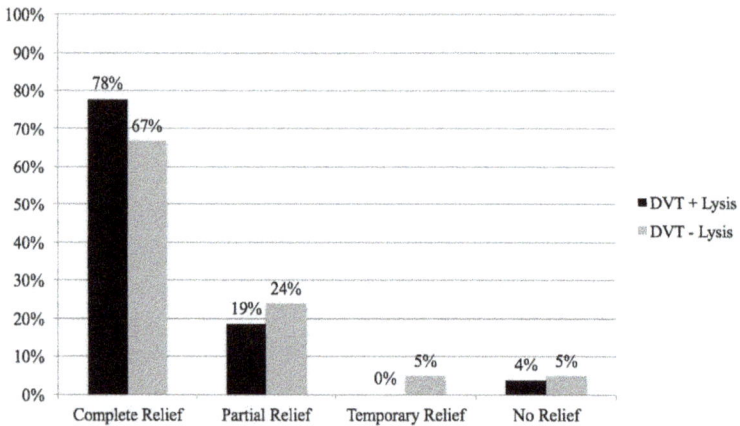

Figure 2. Outcomes with or without preoperative thrombolysis following FRR.

Performance of FRR less than or greater than six weeks after preoperative thrombolysis was not related to FRR outcomes ($p = 0.444$; Figure 3).

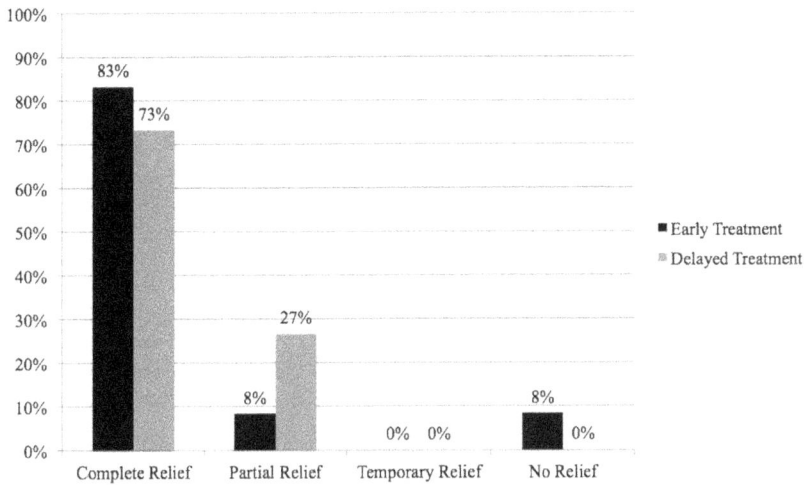

Figure 3. Outcomes after FRR less than or greater than six weeks after presentation.

Whether patients were diagnosed with a DVT or had MCS only was not related to FRR outcomes ($p = 0.796$). No patient had a recurrent DVT. Pneumothorax occurred in 10%. By definition, of the 43 patients who had complete responses, all were able to return to their preoperative occupation or athletic activity and had no residual symptoms. Of the 13 patients who had partial responses, all had mild residual arm swelling but had significant symptomatic improvement and were able to return to their pre-operative occupational or athletic function. Median follow-up was 3.7 months.

By VTOS subclass, 72% of DVT patients and 67% of MCS patients achieved a complete response. Overall, of those with temporary or no response, two patients had chronic axillary vein occlusion after FRR and underwent subsequent venoplasty; one achieved complete response after this while the other demonstrated re-thrombosis and return of symptoms treated with ongoing anticoagulation but does not have functional limitation. The other two patients with temporary or no response had patent axillosubclavian veins on interrogation, but one was diagnosed with chronic regional pain syndrome and the other was found to have severe cervical degenerative disc disease with median and ulnar nerve entrapment.

4. Discussion

In this cohort of VTOS patients, an analysis emphasizing patient-centered and functional outcomes demonstrated that FRR is effective for the treatment of symptoms of VTOS including swelling/discoloration/heaviness, collaterals, and functional impairment. Furthermore, no differences in these outcomes were identified based on use of preoperative thrombolysis or the timing of FRR after thrombolysis in VTOS. Lastly, FRR was found to be effective in treating symptoms associated with MCS.

Historically, outcomes for VTOS have focused on DVT recurrence and axillosubclavian vein patency. In our practice, we have emphasized patient-centered and functional outcomes, as available evidence suggests that most VTOS patients will do well from a DVT recurrence standpoint after FRR, even if venous stenosis or occlusion persists [7]. We did not have any DVT recurrence in this series. Furthermore, Machleder, in his 1993 report, recognized that significant numbers of patients left with chronically occluded veins after FRR would still go on to have excellent symptom relief and functional recovery [7]. Heron et al. in 1991 showed that in 54 patients with spontaneous axillosubclavian thrombosis treated with anticoagulation alone, though 22% of patients had persistent venous occlusion, venous patency did not correlate with symptom resolution [8]. In our practice, we similarly have found that a majority of patients do well symptomatically, often even in the setting of chronically occluded veins, and so patient-reported symptoms, functional restoration, and satisfaction with treatment form the basis for our recommendations after FRR. Thus, we do not routinely interrogate the axillosubclavian vein for patency, though we do so aggressively if the patient is anything other than totally asymptomatic. Our outcomes with this approach to the disease, in addition to how thrombolysis and timing of surgery may affect them, formed the basis for this study.

The timing of FRR for VTOS in patients with DVT who undergo preoperative thrombolysis remains controversial. Machleder initially advocated for delaying surgery as long as three months after thrombolysis to minimize complication risk caused by acute inflammation from DVT and to avoid the thrombogenicity of a recently thrombophlebitic vein [7]. Advocates of thrombolysis followed by immediate surgery remain concerned for rethrombosis prior to FRR [9,10]. Recently, Elixène et al. found that, of patients treated with thrombolysis followed by FRR within 10 days, 100% demonstrated complete resolution of symptoms at a median follow-up of 240 months [11]. Angle et al. similarly reported that early rib resection after thrombolysis is safe and may reduce the risk of rethrombosis during a longer waiting interval [9]. Our data showed that the time to FRR of less than or greater than six weeks after thrombolysis did not statistically significantly impact symptomatic or functional outcomes. Ninety-one percent of patients undergoing FRR within six weeks of thrombolysis achieved symptom resolution, and 100% of those undergoing FRR six weeks or more after thrombolysis achieved symptom resolution. This finding stands in agreement with de León et al., who reported complete remission of symptoms in 95.5% of patients following FRR regardless of the timing of surgery [12].

Alternatively, some advocate anticoagulation only prior to FRR for VTOS, and do not believe that routine preoperative thrombolysis of DVT is necessary. Guzzo et al. compared patients who had thrombolysis prior to FRR with those who had anticoagulation only prior to FRR in a series of 110 procedures [13]. In both cohorts, 91% of patients had symptomatic improvement and venous patency at one year [13]. This finding was substantiated by Sabeti et al., who reported that patients who underwent thrombolysis had a higher rate of venous patency but a similar rate of symptom resolution compared to those who were treated with anticoagulation alone [14]. Despite these findings, anticoagulation with thrombolysis continues to be a more common practice.

In our study, functional outcomes were similar after FRR for both DVT and MCS patients. A number of studies examining FRR for VTOS have included MCS patients without performing separate analyses, and few studies have examined outcomes for these patients specifically. Likes et al. presented a cohort of 19 patients who underwent 20 FRR for MCS. At the date of last follow-up, all patients were symptom-free following surgical intervention [15]. In a subgroup analysis, de León et al. similarly reported an 81% complete symptom resolution rate after FRR for MCS (nine of 11 patients) [12].

Lastly, transaxillary, infraclavicular, and paraclavicular surgical approaches to FRR for VTOS have all been advocated [6,16]. A paraclavicular approach to FRR clearly affords the best exposure of the vein, and this technique makes sense when open venous reconstruction is planned [16]. In our practice, however, we typically perform transaxillary resections for VTOS with the understanding that we will rely on transcatheter venous procedures post-operatively in the minority of patients who do not achieve symptom resolution or functional recovery. We have been able to achieve satisfactory patient-reported outcomes while minimizing post-operative venous interrogation and intervention, and thus have not found a compelling need for aggressive intra-operative venous reconstruction afforded by a paraclavicular approach.

Significant limitations of this study are apparent. This is a retrospective study without randomization, thus selection bias affected the choices of pre-operative thrombolysis and timing of FRR. Because follow-up was guided completely by patient-reported symptoms, there was no consistent long-term follow-up for all patients. Although all patients who achieved satisfactory symptom control were instructed to call with recurrent problems, it is clearly possible that some did not. Thus, while the short 3.7 months follow-up may reflect that many patients did well without residual symptoms or functional limitation and did not seek further care, it may also falsely increase our favorable outcome rate if patients with recurrence chose not to initiate further care. And because our approach did not include universal venous interrogation after FRR, we do not have complete data on post-operative patency or how that may have affected patient-centered outcomes. Finally, as attention to patient-centered outcomes has increased, the availability of instruments to quantify outcomes for diseases such as TOS that manifest with relatively subjective symptoms has increased, and we plan to implement these instruments in future studies of our approach to VTOS.

5. Conclusions

A patient-centered approach to guiding post-FRR testing and intervention is safe and reasonable. Symptom control and return to function are effectively achieved with FRR regardless of preoperative thrombolysis or the timing of surgery after thrombolysis. Additionally, patients with MCS can achieve very good symptom relief after FRR.

Author Contributions: Michael R. Go and Nicolas J. Mouawad conceived and designed the study; Colin P. Ryan and Michael R. Go designed the data collection tools, collected data, analyzed and interpreted data, performed statistical analysis, wrote the manuscript, and critically revised the manuscript; Patrick S. Vaccaro collected data and critically revised the manuscript.

Conflicts of Interest: The authors declare no conflict of interest.

References

1. Peek, J.; Vos, C.G.; Ünlü, Ç.; van de Pavoordt, H.D.W.M.; van den Akker, P.J.; de Vries, J.P.M. Outcome of Surgical Treatment for Thoracic Outlet Syndrome: Systematic Review and Meta-Analysis. *Ann. Vasc. Surg.* **2017**, *40*, 303–326. [CrossRef] [PubMed]
2. Povlsen, B.; Hansson, T.; Povlsen, S.D. Treatment for thoracic outlet syndrome. *Cochrane Database Syst. Rev.* **2014**, *11*, CD007218. [CrossRef] [PubMed]
3. Illig, K.A.; Donahue, D.; Duncan, A.; Freischlag, J.; Gelabert, H.; Johansen, K.; Jordan, S.; Sanders, R.; Thompson, R. Reporting standards of the Society for Vascular Surgery for thoracic outlet syndrome. *J. Vasc. Surg.* **2016**, *64*, 797–802. [CrossRef] [PubMed]
4. Derkash, R.S.; Goldberg, V.M.; Mendelson, H.; Mevicker, R. The results of first rib resection in thoracic outlet syndrome. *Orthopedics* **1981**, *4*, 1025–1029. [PubMed]
5. Degeorges, R.; Reynaud, C.; Becquemin, J.P. Thoracic outlet syndrome surgery: Long-term functional results. *Ann. Vasc. Surg.* **2004**, *18*, 558–565. [CrossRef] [PubMed]
6. Orlando, M.S.; Likes, K.C.; Mirza, S.; Cao, Y.; Cohen, A.; Lum, Y.W.; Reifsnyder, T.; Freischlag, J.A. A decade of excellent outcomes after surgical intervention in 538 patients with thoracic outlet syndrome. *J. Am. Coll. Surg.* **2015**, *220*, 934–939. [CrossRef] [PubMed]
7. Machleder, H.I. Evaluation of a new treatment strategy for Paget-Schroetter syndrome: Spontaneous thrombosis of the axillary-subclavian vein. *J. Vasc. Surg.* **1993**, *17*, 305–315. [CrossRef]
8. Héron, E.; Lozinguez, O.; Emmerich, J.; Laurian, C.; Fiessinger, J.N. Long-term sequelae of spontaneous axillary-subclavian venous thrombosis. *Ann. Intern. Med.* **1999**, *131*, 510–513. [CrossRef] [PubMed]
9. Angle, N.; Gelebert, H.A.; Farooq, M.M.; Ahn, S.; Caswell, D.; Freischlag, J.; Machleder, H.I. Safety and efficacy of early surgical decompression of the thoracicoutlet for Paget-Schroetter syndrome. *Ann. Vasc. Surg.* **2001**, *15*, 37–42. [CrossRef] [PubMed]
10. Urschel, H.C.; Razzuk, M.A. Improved management of the Paget-Schroetter syndrome secondary to thoracic outlet compression. *Ann. Thorac. Surg.* **1991**, *52*, 1217–1221. [CrossRef]
11. Elixène, J.B.; Sadaghianloo, N.; Mousnier, A.; Brizzi, S.; Declemy, S.; Hassen-Khodja, R. Long-term functional outcomes and subclavian vein patency in patients undergoing thoracic outlet surgery for Paget-Schroetter Syndrome. *J. Cardiovasc. Surg.* **2017**, *58*, 451–457.
12. De León, R.A.; Chang, D.C.; Hassoun, H.T.; Black, J.H.; Roseborough, G.S.; Perler, B.A.; Rotellini-Coltvet, L.; Call, D.; Busse, C.; Freischlag, J.A. Multiple treatment algorithms for successful outcomes in venous thoracic outlet syndrome. *Surgery* **2009**, *145*, 500–507. [CrossRef] [PubMed]

13. Guzzo, J.L.; Chang, K.; Demos, J.; Black, J.H.; Freischlag, J.A. Preoperative thrombolysis and venoplasty affords no benefit in patency following first rib resection and scalenectomy for subacute and chronic subclavian vein thrombosis. *J. Vasc. Surg.* **2010**, *52*, 658–662. [CrossRef] [PubMed]
14. Sabeti, S.; Schillinger, M.; Mlekusch, W.; Haumer, M.; Ahmadi, R.; Minar, E. Treatment of subclavian-axillary vein thrombosis: Long-term outcome of anticoagulation versus systemic thrombolysis. *Thromb. Res.* **2002**, *108*, 279–285. [CrossRef]
15. Likes, K.; Rochlin, D.H.; Call, D.; Freischlag, J.A. McCleery syndrome: Etiology and outcome. *Vasc. Endovasc. Surg.* **2014**, *48*, 106–110. [CrossRef] [PubMed]
16. Vemuri, C.; Salehi, P.; Benarroch-Gampel, J.; McLaughlin, L.N.; Thompson, R.W. Diagnosis and treatment of effort-induced thrombosis of the axillary subclavian vein due to venous thoracic outlet syndrome. *J. Vasc. Surg. Venous Lymphat. Disord.* **2016**, *4*, 485–500. [CrossRef] [PubMed]

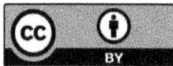

diagnostics

MDPI

Article

A Prospective Evaluation of Duplex Ultrasound for Thoracic Outlet Syndrome in High-Performance Musicians Playing Bowed String Instruments

Garret Adam [1], **Kevin Wang** [2], **Christopher J. Demaree** [3], **Jenny S. Jiang** [4], **Mathew Cheung** [5], **Carlos F. Bechara** [6] and **Peter H. Lin** [1,5,*]

1   Michael E. DeBakey Department of Surgery, Baylor College of Medicine, Houston, TX 77030, USA
2   Department of Medicine, Keck School of Medicine, University of Southern California, Los Angeles, CA 90007, USA
3   Department of Medicine, Tulane University School of Medicine, New Orleans, LA 70112, USA
4   Department of Medicine, University of Texas MD Anderson Cancer Center, Houston, TX 77030, USA
5   Univesity Vascular Associates, Los Angeles, CA 90024, USA
6   Department of Surgery, Stritch School of Medicine, Loyola University Chicago, Maywood, IL 60153, USA
*   Correspondence: plin@bcm.edu; Tel.: +1-713-798-5685

Received: 26 December 2017; Accepted: 22 January 2018; Published: 25 January 2018

Abstract: Thoracic outlet syndrome (TOS) is a neurovascular condition involving the upper extremity, which is known to occur in individuals who perform chronic repetitive upper extremity activities. We prospectively evaluate the incidence of TOS in high-performance musicians who played bowed string musicians. Sixty-four high-performance string instrument musicians from orchestras and professional musical bands were included in the study. Fifty-two healthy volunteers formed an age-matched control group. Bilateral upper extremity duplex scanning for subclavian vessel compression was performed in all subjects. Provocative maneuvers including Elevated Arm Stress Test (EAST) and Upper Limb Tension Test (ULTT) were performed. Abnormal ultrasound finding is defined by greater than 50% subclavian vessel compression with arm abduction, diminished venous waveforms, or arterial photoplethysmography (PPG) tracing with arm abduction. Bowed string instruments performed by musicians in our study included violin (41%), viola (33%), and cello (27%). Positive EAST or ULTT test in the musician group and control group were 44%, and 3%, respectively ($p = 0.03$). Abnormal ultrasound scan with vascular compression was detected in 69% of musicians, in contrast to 15% of control subjects ($p = 0.03$). TOS is a common phenomenon among high-performance bowed string instrumentalists. Musicians who perform bowed string instruments should be aware of this condition and its associated musculoskeletal symptoms.

Keywords: thoracic outlet syndrome; nerve entrapment syndrome; musician; bowed string instrument; violin; viola; cello

1. Introduction

Thoracic outlet syndrome (TOS) is due to the compression of the neurovascular structure in the thoracic inlet, as it commonly affects individuals who perform repetitive upper extremity physical activity. Neurogenic TOS, which is the most common subtype of TOS, often represents a diagnostic challenge for clinicians due in part to a lack of definitive imaging modality as well as non-specific neuromuscular symptoms which may include pain, paresthesia, weakness, fatigue, or tingling sensation of the affected arm. The diagnosis of TOS primarily requires a comprehensive assessment of clinical symptoms as well as physical examination findings. Pertinent findings on the physical examination in patients with TOS can include positive Elevated Arm Stress Test (EAST) and Upper Limb Tension Test (ULTT). Clinical studies have also highlighted an important diagnostic value of duplex ultrasound and photoplethysmography (PPG) which can detect vascular compression with dampened waveform in patients with TOS [1,2].

Individuals who participate in high-level repetitive physical activity involving the upper extremity have an increased risk of developing TOS. Previous reports have linked TOS to high-performance athletes who engaged in repetitive overhead motions, such as baseball pitchers, volleyball players, and swimmers [3–5]. High-performance musicians who play instruments with repetitive arm motions are at risk of developing similar musculoskeletal ailments and nerve entrapment syndromes commonly seen in athletes, with typical examples including carpal tunnel syndrome, ulnar neuropathy, and cubital tunnel syndrome [6–9]. However, studies regarding thoracic outlet syndrome in high-performance musicians remain scarce. We recently reported a case series of professional violinist and violaists who underwent successful first rib resection and scalenectomy for neurogenic TOS [10]. We hypothesize that professional bowed string musicians, who perform musical instruments with repetitive arm motions, have an increased incidence of TOS. In this prospective study, we analyzed possible thoracic outlet syndrome using both physical examinations and ultrasound assessments in high-performance bowed string musicians.

2. Materials and Methods

This was a prospective study of TOS of 64 professional or elite bowed string musicians who were recruited on a volunteer basis from three metropolitan symphony orchestra, two collegiate symphony orchestra, and four professional rock bands. Fifty-two healthy non-musician subjects were also recruited which formed the control group. Inclusion criteria included subjects with a full range of motion of the upper extremities who did not suffer from any musculoskeletal ailments which limited their arm mobility. Exclusion criteria included those with a history of upper extremity injury or orthopedic procedures with movement limitations. Consent was obtained from all participants, and the study was conducted with the approval of institutional review board. The project identification code is IRB# 43529975BYC. The date of approval is 3 March 2012.

Each participant completed a questionnaire related to upper extremity activities in his or her daily routine. Associated symptoms with upper extremity activities were surveyed. Each participant underwent a detailed upper extremity physical exanimation by a board certified vascular surgeon including palpation over scalene triangle and subcoracoid space for localized tenderness. Provocative maneuvers including EAST and ULTT were also performed, and techniques for these provocative maneuvers were based on a previous publication [11].

Duplex ultrasound was performed in each subject by certified vascular ultrasonographers, in which subclavian artery and vein with their respective velocities were recorded. Measurements for each limb were obtained with the head turned 90 degree to abducted contralateral arm. Abnormal scans were defined as ipsilateral compression with greater than 50% increase or decrease in velocity in the subclavian artery or vein on abduction compared to adduction. A portable ultrasound unit SonoSite Edge II (Fujifilm SonoSite, Inc. Bothell, WA, USA) with an 8–5 MHz bandwidth transducer probe was placed in the infraclavicular space, with the vessel imaged in both longitudinal as well as perpendicular fashion to obtain a round cross-sectional image. In all arm positions, the waveforms were recorded as phasic, bidirectional, continuous, minimally continuous, or absent. Images and waveforms were compared between the two groups.

Physiologic assessment of arterial flow variations based on arm position was performed. A PPG sensor was placed in the subject's index finger of the extremity under study in which the corresponding PPG tracings were analyzed using a non-invasive vascular system Flo-Lab 2100-SX2 (Park Medical Electronics, Inc., Aloha, OR, USA). PPG waveforms were interpreted as normal, dampened, or absent. In an identical fashion, arterial flow velocities were obtained at rest and in all positions. Velocities in both resting and provocative positions were recorded and analyzed. The velocity ratio of provocative position to resting position was calculated.

Data were expressed as mean ± standard deviation. Statistical analysis was performed using Fisher's exact test or Pearson's chi-square test in categorical variables. Wilcoxon rank-sum test was used to test for differences in continuous variables. All statistical analysis were performed using a statistical software program (SAS Institute, Cary, NC, USA). Statistical significance was accepted with a *p*-value of less than 0.05.

3. Results

Among the bowed string musicians, there were 26 violinists (41%), 21 violaists (33%), and 14 cellists (27%). No difference is noted with regards to their age and gender distribution between the musician and control groups, which were shown in Table 1. The musician group reported a significantly longer daily repetitive upper extremity activity with a mean of 5.3 ± 2.4 h, which was in contrast to 0.6 ± 0.4 h of daily activity in the control group (p = 0.001). The musicians reported playing musical instruments while control subjects noted computer activity were their respective reasons for daily repetitive upper extremity activity.

Table 1. Baseline demographic information and upper extremity activity.

Characteristics	Musician Group (n = 64)	Control Group (n = 52)	*p*-Value
Age, mean ± SD (years)	35 ± 9.3	28 ± 11.6	NS
Age, range (years)	21–53	19–48	
Gender			
Male	28 (44%)	25 (48%)	
Female	36 (56%)	27 (52%)	NS
Bowed string instrument played			
Violin	26 (41%)	N/A	
Viola	21 (33%)	N/A	
Cello	17 (27%)	N/A	
Duration of daily upper extremity repetitive activity (hour)	5.3 ± 2.4	0.6 ± 0.4	0.001

NS means non-significant.

Results of physical examination with regards to localized tenderness on palpation in the scalene triangle and subcoracoid space were displayed in Table 2. Twenty-two musicians (34%) experienced localized tenderness to palpation in the scalene triangle, in contrast to one control subject (2%) with localized scalene triangle tenderness. Greater proportion of these musicians showed a left sided scalene triangle tenderness compared to right (25% vs. 9%, p = 0.04). Three musicians (5%) and one control subject (2%) developed subcoracoid space tenderness (NS). Combining the results of scalene triangle and subcoracoid space tenderness, the musician group had a greater positive exam for localized tenderness compared to the control group (39% vs. 4%, p = 0.01). Comparison of provocative maneuvers between the two groups were shown in Table 3. Eighteen musicians (28%) had positive EAST and 17 musicians (27%) had positive ULTT in response to provocative maneuvers, in contrast to two control subjects (4%) to each of these maneuvers (p = 0.04). A greater tendency of left arm positive EAST or ULTT than right arm is observed in the musician group. Combining the results of EAST and ULTT assessments, the overall positive provocative maneuvers in the musician and control group were 44% and 6%, respectively (p = 0.03).

Table 2. Comparison of physical examination between the musician and control groups.

Test Performed	Musician Group (n = 64)	Control Group (n = 52)	p-Value
Physical Examination (Localized Tenderness on Palpation)			
Scalene triangle tenderness (right)	6 (9%)	1 (2%)	
Scalene triangle tenderness (left)	16 (25%)	0	
Overall scalene triangle tenderness	22 (34%)	1 (2%)	0.03
Physical Examination (Localized Tenderness on Palpation)			
Subcoracoid space (right)	1 (2%)	1 (2%)	
Subcoracoid space (left)	2 (3%)	0	
Overall subcoracoid space tenderness	3 (5%)	1 (2%)	NS
Overall positive exam for localized tenderness	25 (39%)	2 (4%)	0.03

Table 3. Comparison of provocative maneuvers between the musician and control groups.

Test Performed	Musician Group (n = 64)	Control Group (n = 52)	p-Value
Provocative Maneuvers			
Positive EAST (right)	7 (11%)	1 (2%)	
Positive EAST (left)	11 (17%)	1 (2%)	
Overall Positive EAST	18 (28%)	2 (4%)	0.04
Provocative Maneuvers			
Positive ULTT (right)	5 (8%)	2 (4%)	
Positive ULTT (left)	12 (19%)	0	
Overall Positive ULTT	17 (27%)	2 (4%)	0.04
Overall positive provocative maneuvers	28 (44%)	3 (6%)	0.03

Subclavian vessel compression based on ultrasound assessment in the musician group and control groups revealed 47% versus 12%, respectively (Table 4, $p = 0.04$). The laterality of subclavian vessel compression in these groups were shown in Table 4. Among the musicians, there is a greater subclavian vessel compression in the left arm compared to the right side (36% vs. 22%). No difference in laterality of subclavian vessel compression was noted in the control group. Venous duplex waveforms were examined with arm abduction while the head was rotated either ipsilaterally or contralaterally from the abducted limb. In the musician group, head turned away from an abducted arm with resultant loss of bi-directional flow or diminution of normal phasicity occurred in 36% of subjects ($n = 23$), in contrast to 8% of the control subjects ($n = 4$, $p < 0.03$). When the head was turned toward an abducted arm, loss of bi-directional flow or diminution of normal phasicity occurred in 22% of musicians ($n = 14$) compared to 6% of the control subjects ($n = 2$). Overall abnormal venous waveform with arm abduction was noted in 56% of musicians compared to 13% of control subjects ($p = 0.03$). Arterial PPG tracings were analyzed with arm abduction while the head was positioned either toward or away from an abducted limb. Abnormal PPG results were defined by dampened or absent tracing, or provocative position to resting position velocity ratios greater than 2.0. Diminished or absent arterial PPG tracing with arm abduction was noted in 25% of musicians in contrast to 6% of control subjects ($p = 0.04$). Overall abnormal ultrasound or PPG test was found in 69% of musicians in contrast to 15% of control subjects ($p = 0.03$). Among these musicians, abnormal arterial PPG tracing or venous duplex waveform were detected in 56% of violists or violaists compared to 18% of cellists ($p = 0.03$). There is a statistical difference in arterial and venous flow anomalies based on PPG or ultrasound assessment in the left arm compared to the right arm in violinists and violaists ($p = 0.04$). There was no difference in the arm laterality with respected to abnormal PPG or waveforms in cellists. Subjects with positive provocative maneuvers were analyzed with abnormal ultrasound or PPG results in both musician and control group, and these results were shown in Table 5. In the musician group, there were 23 subjects (36%) with both positive provocative maneuver test and abnormal ultrasound results which was in contrast to three subjects (6%, $p = 0.03$) in the control group. When we analyzed the laterality of provocative maneuvers versus abnormal ultrasound or PPG results, there was no statistical difference between these variables in either the musician or control subjects.

Table 4. Comparison of ultrasound and PPG evaluation between the musician and control groups.

Test Performed	Musician Group (n = 64)	Control Group (n = 52)	p-Value
Ultrasound Evaluation			
Subclavian vessel compression with arm abduction	30 (47%)	6 (12%)	0.04
Abnormal venous waveforms			
90° arm abduction, head turned contralateral	23 (36%)	4 (8%)	
90° arm abduction, head turned ipsilateral	14 (22%)	3 (6%)	
Overall abnormal venous waveform result	36 (56%)	7 (13%)	0.03
Abnormal arterial PPG tracing			
90° arm abduction, head turned contralateral	11 (17%)	2 (4%)	
90° arm abduction, head turned ipsilateral	7 (11%)	1 (2%)	
Overall abnormal arterial PPG tracing	16 (25%)	3 (6%)	0.04
Overall abnormal ultrasound or PPG test	44 (69%)	8 (15%)	0.03

Table 5. Assessment of positive provocative maneuvers with the presence of abnormal ultrasound or PPG results.

Diagnostic Study	Musician Group (n = 64)			Control Group (n = 52)		
	Positive EAST (n = 18)	Positive ULTT (n = 17)	Overall Positive Provocative Maneuvers (n = 28)	Positive EAST (n = 2)	Positive ULTT (n = 2)	Overall Positive Provocative Maneuvers (n = 3)
Subclavian vessel compression (>50%)	6 (9%)	4 (6%)	10 (36%)	1 (2%)	1 (2%)	2 (3%)
Abnormal venous waveforms	10 (16%)	7 (11%)	14 (50%)	1 (2%)	1 (2%)	2 (3%)
Abnormal arterial PPG tracing	7 (11%)	5 (8%)	11 (39%)	0	0	0
Overall abnormal ultrasound or PPG test	15 (23%)	14 (22%)	23 (36%) *	2 (3%)	2 (3%)	3 (6%) *

% = percentage of patient is calculated based on the total number of patients in the musician or control group respectively. * p = 0.03 when compared between the musician and control group.

4. Discussion

High-performance musicians who perform instruments with repetitive physical motion can endure significant musculoskeletal strain and physical stress with time. Although multiple physical ailments related to nerve entrapment and joint disorders have been described in elite musicians [7,8,12–15], published reports of TOS in these musical instrumentalists remain scarce. The findings of our study are notable as it represents the first prospective evaluation demonstrating TOS is common among elite bowed string musicians, particularly violinists and violists, based on both physical examination as well as ultrasound and PPG assessment.

Although TOS was first described in the early 19th century by Sir Astley Cooper, who treated a patient with a subclavian artery aneurysm caused by first rib compression [16], this condition has continued to pose a significant diagnostic challenge for clinicians due in part to its uncommon incidence, as well as a lack of a single diagnostic test to confirm this condition unequivocally. The Consortium for Outcomes Research and Education of Thoracic Outlet Syndrome recently proposed a preliminary set of diagnostic criteria for TOS [17]. A subsequent updated reporting standard for TOS was published by the Society for Vascular Surgery which include: symptoms of pathology at the thoracic outlet, symptoms of nerve compression, the absence of other pathology potentially explaining the symptoms, and a positive scalene muscle injection test [11]. While these guidelines are useful in differentiating various musculoskeletal ailments from TOS, there still remain many limitations. For instance, these standards recommend the use of scalene muscle injection for diagnostic evaluation, which is a highly specialized procedure that may not be readily available in many clinical practices. Many patients may be unwilling to undergo this invasive test for diagnostic evaluation. Additionally, these guidelines do not include ultrasound or PPG assessment for analyzing subclavian vessel compression. With these considerations in mind we, therefore, adopted more practical diagnostic criteria in our study by incorporating pertinent physical examinations, provocative maneuvers, and ultrasound assessment in our volunteer subjects. We also correlated positive provocative maneuvers with abnormal ultrasound findings for subclavian vessel compression to detect the incidence of TOS between the musician group and the control subjects.

Clinical studies utilizing duplex ultrasound to detect subclavian vessel compression in patients with TOS have reported varied results [1,2,18–21]. Orlando et al., reported their experience of 143 TOS patients who underwent bilateral preoperative duplex ultrasound prior to first rib resection and scalenectomy, and significant flow abnormality was defined as greater than 50% flow reduction with arm abduction. The authors found abnormal subclavian vessel compression in 49% of patients [20]. Demondion et al. used B-mode ultrasound to evaluate thoracic outlet arterial compression in 28 patients with TOS as well as 44 normal individuals, and reported six of the 44 volunteers (14.6%) had arterial stenosis greater than 70% when the arm is extended at 170° [18]. The finding of subclavian vessel compression in healthy individuals has also been reported by several researchers. A recent study from the University of Michigan examined bilateral duplex scans in 50 healthy volunteers and found abnormal duplex scans by either PPG waveforms or velocities in 60% of veins and 30% of arteries with significant variability with arm positioning [1]. The authors reported that dampened or absent PPG tracings are more reliable indicators of hemodynamically-significant vascular compression compared to flow velocities, as the PPG tracings are truly reflective of flow-restrictive changes occurring during positional changes. Colon et al., analyzed PPG finger tracing in 115 health subjects and noted that 44% of them experience severe arterial flow reduction when the arm is abducted in 120° position [2]. Similarly, Longley et al., evaluated 20 normal individuals along with 16 patients with TOS using Doppler ultrasound. They defined significant arterial compression as doubling of peak systolic velocity or complete flow cessation in hyperabduction, while venous abnormality as complete cessation of blood flow or loss of respiratory phasicity with arm hyperabduction. The authors found that 20% of the volunteers had abnormal arterial compression and 10% had significant venous compression with arm abduction [19]. Lastly, Rohrer et al., performed ultrasound evaluation in 46 volunteers including 19 major league baseball pitchers, 16 non-pitching major league players, and 11 non-athlete controls for thoracic outlet compression in the throwing position. They found 56% of these subjects had significant subclavian and axillary with blood pressure decrease of greater than 20 mm Hg. The authors concluded that repetitive upper extremity trauma of the throwing motion can the principle culprit of the arterial compression [21]. These studies all underscored a common observation that subclavian vessel compression can occur in healthy asymptomatic individuals. Furthermore, the degree of thoracic outlet vessel compression can be influenced by the provocative arm position, and results of subclavian vessel compression may vary based on the method of analysis.

In our study, we defined abnormal scan as vessel compression of greater than 50% or reduced PPG waveforms with arm abduction. We found abnormal ultrasound scan by either PPG waveforms or velocities was detected in 69% of musicians, in contrast to 15% of volunteer subjects (Table 4). Those with positive provocative maneuvers with either EAST or ULTT in the musician and control groups were 44% and 6%, respectively (Table 3). Combining the findings of abnormal ultrasound scan and positive provocative maneuver tests, the diagnosis of TOS is made in 37% of musicians, in contrast to 6% of control subjects (Table 5). Among bowed string musicians, abnormal ultrasound scans were more commonly detected in violists and violists compared to cellists, which were 56% and 18% respectively. Although viola is a heavier instrument compared to violin, we did not find difference in subclavian vessel compression base on ultrasound assessment between violinists and violists. We postulate that, because violin and viola are similar string instruments which are positioned above the clavicle and stabilized by the left hand in an elevated position, this creates considerable physical strain to the thoracic outlet as well as the left arm. In contrast, a cello is a string instrument positioned on the ground which does not incur physical strain to the clavicle or requires the musician to maintain the musical instrument in an elevated position.

Reports of musculoskeletal injures and nerve entrapment syndromes have been previously reported in bowed string musicians [7,15,22–24]. In a study analyzing 76 adolescent string musicians from the West Australian Youth Orchestras, 73.5% of the surveyed violinists reported upper extremity musculoskeletal symptoms with pain or paresthesia involving the shoulder, elbow, or wrist joint [25]. In two review articles which analyzed 342 and 117 musicians, respectively, researchers reported a high incidence of compression neuropathy involving the left arm among violinists, particularly left ulnar neuropathy at the elbow due to left forearm supination with wrist flexion while playing the instrument [6,8]. This elbow inward supination is necessary when playing the G or D strings, which are located on the left outer region of the strings. Another study has similarly documented ulnar nerve entrapment syndrome involving the left elbow among violinists, as evidenced by abnormal nerve conduction and electromyography studies [15]. Our study revealed a greater incidence of ultrasound abnormality and positive provocative maneuver tests in the left arm compared to the right arm among the violinists or violists, which underscores the physical stress endured by the left upper extremity in these musicians. Researchers have even coined the term "the droopy shoulder syndrome" to characterize an abnormal contour of the cervical and thoracic spines among violin players, which is attributed in part to chronic clavicle pressure exertion by the stringed instrument pressed against the left clavicle [26]. Using an infrared thermographic imaging, Clemente et al. documented left temporomandibular joint disorders in elite violists with muscle hyperactivity of the head and cervical muscles, and the authors postulated the temporomandibular disorder was due to strained shoulder and neck postures during long musical performances by bowed string instrumentalists [22]. Several reports have similarly described a high incidence of musculoskeletal ailments including functional dystonia involving upper extremities, due in part to abnormal posture and prolonged musculoskeletal strains among bowed string instrumentalists [7,13,15,23]. Other researchers have suggested that the neck position of violinists while playing may predispose them to cervical radiculopathy [12,27–29]. Taking into consideration these published reports, we speculate the physical strain experienced by high-performance bowed string musicians has contributed in part to the pathogenesis of various musculoskeletal disorders and nerve entrapment syndromes of the upper extremities, including TOS.

There are inevitably several weaknesses worth considering. Abnormal duplex ultrasound with subclavian vessel compression was not an infrequent finding as we detected this occurrence in 15% of our healthy volunteers. Consequently, critics may challenge the comparative value regarding the diagnostic sensitivity of TOS in these elite musicians when compared to the control subjects. Additionally, TOS is a clinical condition which encompasses a myriad of neurovascular compressive symptoms, and its diagnosis cannot be based on sonographic evidence of neurovascular compression alone. Although we utilized provocative maneuvers, such as the EAST and ULTT, to elicit symptoms of TOS, the reliability of these provocative physical tests combined with abnormal ultrasound assessment has not been validated with proven diagnostic sensitivity for TOS. In spite of these study limitations, our study underscored a causative relation between high-performance bowed string instrumentalists and TOS.

In conclusion, our study showed a high prevalence of neurovascular compression in elite stringed instrumentalists based on duplex ultrasound evaluation compared to control subjects. The abnormal ultrasound finding also correlates with provocative maneuvers. The finding of this study provides an important diagnostic insight regarding neuromuscular strain caused by chronic repetitive upper extremity physical motion in high-performance musicians. Clinicians should have a heightened level of diagnostic awareness for TOS when treating patients with thoracic outlet strain who are high-performance bowed string musical instrumentalists.

Acknowledgments: This study was supported in part by a research grant from Vascular Institute of Texas (grant #232342).

Author Contributions: Garret Adam and Peter H. Lin conceived and designed the experiments. Garret Adam, Kevin Wang, Christopher J. Demaree, Jenny S. Jiang, Mathew Cheung, Carlos F. Bechara, and Peter H. Lin, performed the experiments; Garret Adam, Kevin Wang, Christopher J. Demaree, Jenny S. Jiang, Mathew Cheung,

Carlos F. Bechara, and Peter H. Lin analyzed the data; Garret Adam, Kevin Wang, Christopher J. Demaree, Jenny S. Jiang, Mathew Cheung, Carlos F. Bechara, and Peter H. Lin contributed the analysis; Garret Adam, Kevin Wang, Christopher J. Demaree, Jenny S. Jiang., M.C., Carlos F. Bechara, and Peter H. Lin contributed the manuscript.

Conflicts of Interest: The authors declare no conflict of interest.

References

1. Chen, H.; Doornbos, N.; Williams, K.; Criado, E. Physiologic variations in venous and arterial hemodynamics in response to postural changes at the thoracic outlet in normal volunteers. *Ann. Vasc. Surg.* **2014**, *28*, 1583–1588. [CrossRef] [PubMed]
2. Colon, E.; Westdorp, R. Vascular compression in the thoracic outlet. Age dependent normative values in noninvasive testing. *J. Cardiovasc. Surg.* **1988**, *29*, 166–171.
3. Chandra, V.; Little, C.; Lee, J.T. Thoracic outlet syndrome in high-performance athletes. *J. Vasc. Surg.* **2014**, *60*, 1012–1017. [CrossRef] [PubMed]
4. McCarthy, W.J.; Yao, J.S.; Schafer, M.F.; Nuber, G.; Flinn, W.R.; Blackburn, D.; Suker, J.R. Upper extremity arterial injury in athletes. *J. Vasc. Surg.* **1989**, *9*, 317–327. [CrossRef]
5. Shutze, W.; Richardson, B.; Shutze, R.; Tran, K.; Dao, A.; Ogola, G.O.; Young, A.; Pearl, G. Midterm and long-term follow-up in competitive athletes undergoing thoracic outlet decompression for neurogenic thoracic outlet syndrome. *J. Vasc. Surg.* **2017**, *66*, 1798–1805. [CrossRef] [PubMed]
6. Charness, M.E.; Ross, M.H.; Shefner, J.M. Ulnar neuropathy and dystonic flexion of the fourth and fifth digits: Clinical correlation in musicians. *Muscle Nerve* **1996**, *19*, 431–437. [CrossRef] [PubMed]
7. Lederman, R.J. Neuromuscular problems in musicians. *Neurologist* **2002**, *8*, 163–174. [CrossRef] [PubMed]
8. Lederman, R.J. Focal peripheral neuropathies in instrumental musicians. *Phys. Med. Rehabil. Clin. N. Am.* **2006**, *17*, 761–779. [CrossRef] [PubMed]
9. Wilson, R.J.; Watson, J.T.; Lee, D.H. Nerve entrapment syndromes in musicians. *Clin. Anat.* **2014**, *27*, 861–865. [CrossRef] [PubMed]
10. Demaree, C.J.; Wang, K.; Lin, P.H. Thoracic outlet syndrome affecting high-performance musicians playing bowed string instruments. *Vascular* **2017**, *25*, 329–332. [CrossRef] [PubMed]
11. Illig, K.A.; Donahue, D.; Duncan, A.; Freischlag, J.; Gelabert, H.; Johansen, K.; Jordan, S.; Sanders, R.; Thompson, R. Reporting standards of the Society for Vascular Surgery for thoracic outlet syndrome. *J. Vasc. Surg.* **2016**, *64*, e23–e35. [CrossRef] [PubMed]
12. Bird, H.A. Overuse syndrome in musicians. *Clin. Rheumatol.* **2013**, *32*, 475–479. [CrossRef] [PubMed]
13. Chamagne, P. Functional dystonia in musicians: Rehabilitation. *Hand Clin.* **2003**, *19*, 309–316. [CrossRef]
14. Lahme, A.; Eibl, I.; Reichl, F.X. Typical musculoskeletal patterns in upper string players with neck and arm problems. *Med. Probl. Perform. Artist.* **2014**, *29*, 241–242.
15. Lee, H.S.; Park, H.Y.; Yoon, J.O.; Kim, J.S.; Chun, J.M.; Aminata, I.W.; Cho, W.J.; Jeon, I.H. Musicians' medicine: Musculoskeletal problems in string players. *Clin. Orthop. Surg.* **2013**, *5*, 155–160. [CrossRef] [PubMed]
16. Gergoudis, R.; Barnes, R.W. Thoracic outlet arterial compression: Prevalence in normal persons. *Angiology* **1980**, *31*, 538–541. [CrossRef] [PubMed]
17. Illig, K.A. *Thoracic Outlet Syndrome*; Thompson, R.W., Freischlag, J.A., Eds.; Springer Science and Business Media: New York, NY, USA, 2014.
18. Demondion, X.; Vidal, C.; Herbinet, P.; Gautier, C.; Duquesnoy, B.; Cotten, A. Ultrasonographic assessment of arterial cross-sectional area in the thoracic outlet on postural maneuvers measured with power Doppler ultrasonography in both asymptomatic and symptomatic populations. *J. Ultrasound Med.* **2006**, *25*, 217–224. [CrossRef] [PubMed]
19. Longley, D.G.; Yedlicka, J.W.; Molina, E.J.; Schwabacher, S.; Hunter, D.W.; Letourneau, J.G. Thoracic outlet syndrome: Evaluation of the subclavian vessels by color duplex sonography. *AJR Am. J. Roentgenol.* **1992**, *158*, 623–630. [CrossRef] [PubMed]
20. Orlando, M.S.; Likes, K.C.; Mirza, S.; Cao, Y.; Cohen, A.; Lum, Y.W.; Freischlag, J.A. Preoperative Duplex Scanning is a Helpful Diagnostic Tool in Neurogenic Thoracic Outlet Syndrome. *Vasc. Endovasc. Surg.* **2016**, *50*, 29–32. [CrossRef] [PubMed]

21. Rohrer, M.J.; Cardullo, P.A.; Pappas, A.M.; Phillips, D.A.; Wheeler, H.B. Axillary artery compression and thrombosis in throwing athletes. *J. Vasc. Surg.* **1990**, *11*, 761–768. [CrossRef]
22. Clemente, M.; Coimbra, D.; Silva, A.; Aguiar Branco, C.; Pinho, J.C. Application of Infrared Thermal Imaging in a Violinist with Temporomandibular Disorder. *Med. Probl. Perform. Artist.* **2015**, *30*, 251–254.
23. Lederman, R.J. Neuromuscular and musculoskeletal problems in instrumental musicians. *Muscle Nerve* **2003**, *27*, 549–561. [CrossRef] [PubMed]
24. Robinson, B.S.; Kincaid, A.E. Repetitive motion in perception of tactile sensation in the fingers of string players. *Percept. Mot. Skills* **2004**, *99*, 1171–1183. [CrossRef] [PubMed]
25. Vinci, S.; Smith, A.; Ranelli, S. Selected Physical Characteristics and Playing-Related Musculoskeletal Problems in Adolescent String Instrumentalists. *Med. Probl. Perform. Artist.* **2015**, *30*, 143–151.
26. Swift, T.R.; Nichols, F.T. The droopy shoulder syndrome. *Neurology* **1984**, *34*, 212–215. [CrossRef] [PubMed]
27. Leijnse, J.N.; Rietveld, A.B. Left shoulder pain in a violinist, related to extensor tendon adhesions in a small scar on the back of the wrist. *Clin. Rheumatol.* **2013**, *32*, 501–506. [CrossRef] [PubMed]
28. Rietveld, A.B.; Leijnse, J.N. Focal hand dystonia in musicians: A synopsis. *Clin. Rheumatol.* **2013**, *32*, 481–486. [CrossRef] [PubMed]
29. Baltopoulos, P.; Tsintzos, C.; Prionas, G.; Tsironi, M. Exercise-induced scalenus syndrome. *Am. J. Sports Med.* **2008**, *36*, 369–374. [CrossRef] [PubMed]

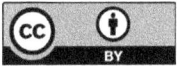

diagnostics

MDPI

Review

Diagnosing Thoracic Outlet Syndrome: Current Approaches and Future Directions

Sebastian Povlsen [1,*] and Bo Povlsen [2]

[1] King's College Hospital NHS Foundation Trust, Denmark Hill, London SE5 9RS, UK
[2] London Hand Clinic, London Bridge Hospital, London SE1 2PR, UK; bo@manusmedical.com
*   Correspondence: seb.povlsen@gmail.com; Tel.: +44-797-964-7073

Received: 19 February 2018; Accepted: 15 March 2018; Published: 20 March 2018

Abstract: The diagnosis of thoracic outlet syndrome (TOS) has long been a controversial and challenging one. Despite common presentations with pain in the neck and upper extremity, there are a host of presenting patterns that can vary within and between the subdivisions of neurogenic, venous, and arterial TOS. Furthermore, there is a plethora of differential diagnoses, from peripheral compressive neuropathies, to intrinsic shoulder pathologies, to pathologies at the cervical spine. Depending on the subdivision of TOS suspected, diagnostic investigations are currently of varying importance, necessitating high dependence on good history taking and clinical examination. Investigations may add weight to a diagnosis suspected on clinical grounds and suggest an optimal management strategy, but in this changing field new developments may alter the role that diagnostic investigations play. In this article, we set out to summarise the diagnostic approach in cases of suspected TOS, including the importance of history taking, clinical examination, and the role of investigations at present, and highlight the developments in this field with respect to all subtypes. In the future, we hope that novel diagnostics may be able to stratify patients according to the exact compressive mechanism and thereby suggest more specific treatments and interventions.

Keywords: thoracic outlet syndrome; neurogenic; venous; arterial; diagnosis; clinical; neurography; diffusion tensor imaging; ultrasound; dynamic CT angiography

---

1. Introduction

Since its inception in 1956 by Peet et al. [1], thoracic outlet syndrome (TOS) has been used to refer to a constellation of symptoms resulting from neurovascular compression at the thoracic outlet, usually resulting in some combination of pain in the neck and upper extremity, weakness, sensory loss, paraesthesias, swelling, and discoloration [2]. The exact constellation of signs and symptoms depends on the exact structures being compressed, but the common symptoms of pain can result from either damage to the subclavian vein, subclavian artery, or different parts of the brachial plexus [3]. Classification systems have used these anatomical structures to subdivide TOS into venous TOS (VTOS), arterial TOS (ATOS), and neurogenic TOS (NTOS). Although diagnosis of any subtype of TOS can prove challenging, the diagnosis of NTOS is particularly difficult due to the branching anatomy of the brachial plexus leading to different constellations of pain, sensory disturbance, and weakness depending on the exact parts being compressed. This perhaps can be exemplified by the fact that many classification systems include a further subcategory of "disputed TOS", where a diagnosis of NTOS is uncertain (perhaps due to the lack of supporting nerve conduction studies) but where the symptomatology is consistent with it [4]. This subdivision is losing its basis in some cases [5]. The difficulty and lack of clarity on the subject of TOS has been acknowledged by the Society for Vascular Surgery [5] from the point of view of both diagnostic criteria and a lack of evidence-based treatment after findings from a Cochrane Collaboration review [6]. Whilst the contribution of imaging and other investigations is variable in diagnosing TOS, the clinical acumen of the practicing physician or surgeon remains key to differentiating the variable presentations of TOS with the numerous potential differential diagnoses of pain in the upper extremity. Here we aim to summarise the diagnostic approach in cases of possible TOS and discuss developments in the field.

2. History

Good clinical acumen always begins with accurate history taking. The common theme to all presentations of TOS is the presence of pain. Questioning should focus on the precise distribution of the pain, its character, and what activities exacerbate the pain. The associated symptomatology should also be sought, as well as the resulting functional limitation experienced by the patient. A summary of findings from the history can be found in Table 1.

Table 1. History and examination features in ATOS, VTOS, and NTOS.

TOS Subtype	History	Examination
ATOS	Claudication/rest pain of upper limb, excluding shoulder/neck Numbness, coolness, pallor	Raynaud's phenomenon Upper limb ischaemia, digital ulceration, peripheral embolisation Pulsatile mass ± bruit on auscultation Blood pressure differential >20 mmHg Positive EAST, ULTT, Adson's test
VTOS	Deep pain on movement or rest pain in upper limb, chest, shoulder Swelling and cyanotic discoloration	Upper limb swelling Cyanosis Positive EAST, ULTT, Adson's test
NTOS	Pain in neck, trapezius, shoulder, arm, chest, occipital headache Variable pattern upper limb weakness, numbness, paraesthesias	Tenderness on palpation: scalene triangle, subcoracoid space Upper plexus (C5-C7): sensory disturbance of arm. Weakness/atrophy of deltoid, biceps, brachialis Lower plexus (C8-T1): sensory disturbance ulnar forearm & hand. Weakness/atrophy of small muscles of the hand, weak wrist & finger flexion Positive EAST, ULTT, Adson's test

The distribution of pain can be very wide in NTOS, but commonly occurs in the neck, trapezius, shoulder, arm, and in some cases also manifests as chest pain and occipital headache. The pain should be non-radicular in nature and be present during activities, where it may limit function, as well as at rest. Paraesthesias can be widespread in the upper extremity and fingers. Non-specific descriptions include heaviness with movements above the shoulder, referring to the weakness of the affected muscle groups [7]. Once this is suspected, history taking may enable one to separate whether the upper or lower parts of the brachial plexus are more involved, with lower plexus (C8-T1) resulting in symptoms in the ulnar forearm and hand, as well as the axillary and anterior shoulder region. Upper plexus compression (C5-C7) results in more supraclavicular symptomatology, with radiations to the chest, periscapular region, and the head and in the distribution of the radial nerve [2]. History should also focus on potential differential diagnoses. If radicular pain is present, cervical radiculopathy should be suspected [8]. Carpal tunnel syndrome and cubital tunnel syndrome, meanwhile, should be suspected if pain and paraesthesia is confined solely to the distribution of the median and ulnar nerves distal to the point of compression in the carpal and cubital tunnels, respectively [9,10]. However, it must be remembered that these may co-exist with a diagnosis of TOS [11].

VTOS will also present with pain of the upper extremity, which may also involve the chest and shoulder. However, this is typically a "deeper" pain and one that is worse with activity. Significant associated symptoms include swelling and cyanotic discoloration of the upper extremity [12]. Sometimes, a presentation will be due to intermittent compression at the costoclavicular junction, in which case it can be aggravated or can present thrombosis of the subclavian vein (Paget–Schroetter syndrome), in which case the symptoms may be more constant and the swelling and discoloration more prominent [2].

Finally, whilst ATOS will also present with a non-radicular pain of the upper extremity, prominent features also include numbness, coolness, and pallor. Distinguishing its distribution from NTOS, pain is rarely present in the shoulder or neck [11]. Claudication may be present, but pain may also be present at rest but worsened by elevating the arms above the head. The symptoms may be intermittent initially due to compression of the subclavian artery by a cervical rib, manifesting as intermittent pain and Raynaud's phenomenon, before complications arising from arterial damage occur (such as aneurysm, thrombosis, and critical limb ischaemia) [2].

It is becoming increasingly recognised that high-level repetitive physical activity involving the upper extremity may put individuals at risk for development of thoracic outlet syndrome. Indeed, in one centre >40% of patients requiring first rib resection and scalenectomy for NTOS relief were competitive athletes [13]. This risk also appears to extend to the vascular subtypes of TOS, where such events may be antecedents for effort-induced thrombosis [14]. Although cases of thoracic outlet syndrome in musicians have been documented [15], until now it had not been rigorously studied. A recent paper in this journal [16] prospectively evaluated 64 high-performance string instrument musicians and 52 healthy age-matched controls. They found positive elevated arm stress test (EAST) or upper limb tension test (ULTT) in 44% of musicians compared with 3% in the control group. Abnormal ultrasound scan with vascular compressions was detected in 69% of musicians versus 15% of controls. Interestingly, they also noted abnormal ultrasound scans with vascular compression were more commonly noted in violinists and viola players than cellists. Furthermore, in violinists and viola players, the left arm, which is elevated to hold up the instrument, was more commonly affected than the right bow-holding hand. This underscores the theory that it is the overhead repetitive-strain aspect of these activities that predisposes to thoracic outlet syndrome. Longitudinal studies of such patient groups would be useful to assess the likelihood of these findings progressing into clinically significant thoracic outlet syndrome requiring surgery. In the meantime, such pre-disposing factors should be ascertained in the history.

3. Examination

By this point in the consultation, a list of differential diagnoses including TOS may start to form. The purpose of clinical examination is to refute some and give weight to others. The general approach to a full evaluation should include a general inspection of the patient with attention to the affected limb in comparison to the contralateral limb, an examination of the cervical spine and neck including the scalene triangle, an examination of the shoulder, a full neurological examination of the upper limbs, a peripheral vascular examination, and the performance of provocative manoeuvres [5]. A summary of examination findings can be found in Table 1.

General inspection should focus on the asymmetry between the affected and contralateral limb. Signs of swelling and cyanotic discoloration may be in keeping with VTOS, whereas the observable Raynaud's phenomenon, upper limb ischaemia, digital ulceration, and signs of peripheral embolisation may be more in keeping with ATOS [2]. NTOS on the other hand may manifest with muscular atrophy, although this is rare—pay attention to the thenar eminence, hypothenar eminence, and the interossei [17]. A clinician should also look for signs of trauma to the chest, clavicle, shoulder, and ribs, which might lead to pathological compression at the thoracic outlet [5].

Examination of the neck, cervical spine, and shoulder should include palpation of the reported sites of pain for tenderness. Palpation at possible sites of compression, such as the supraclavicular scalene triangle or subcoracoid pectoralis minor insertion site, may reproduce symptoms in NTOS [5]. If intrinsic pathology of the shoulder itself is suspected, such as subacromial impingement, adhesive capsulitis or rotator cuff injuries, a full orthopaedic examination of the shoulder should be carried out with Hawkins test positive in impingement [18], adhesive capsulitis resulting in pain in both passive and active movements in all directions [19], and rotator cuff injuries resulting in weakness of the supraspinatus, the infraspinatus, the teres minor, and the subscapularis [20]. Weakness in these respective muscle groups can be tested individually with the Jobe test in which the patient experiences weakness to restricted elevation with the patient's arms at 90° of abduction and internally rotated, the hornblower's test in which the patient experiences weakness in restricted external rotation of the shoulder with the arm held at 90° of abduction and the elbow flexed to 90°, and the lift-off test in which the patient experiences weakness when the dorsum of the hand is placed against the patient's lumbar spine and is then instructed to move the hand away from the back in a perpendicular plane against resistance [21].

A peripheral neurological examination should assess the tone, power, reflexes, and sensation of the affected limb in comparison with the contralateral limb. The distribution of weakness, numbness, and paraesthesias may be variable. Suspicion of the upper brachial plexus (C5-C7) involvement is suggested by sensory disturbance of the arm and weakness and atrophy of the deltoid, biceps, and brachialis muscles. Lower plexus (C8-T1) involvement is suspected by weakness in the small muscles of the hand and weakness of wrist and finger flexion. Sensory loss may be more confined to the ulnar forearm and hand [22]. In reality, 85–90% of cases of NTOS may present with a combination of upper and lower plexus involvement [23]. A key part of the examination at this stage is to try and exclude peripheral compressive neuropathies such as carpal tunnel syndrome and cubital tunnel syndrome. Carpal tunnel syndrome will have sensory disturbance confined to the distribution of the median nerve and tinel's and phalen's tests may be positive, with sensitivities of 67% and 85% and specificities of 68% and 89%, respectively [24]. The sensory disturbance in cubital tunnel syndrome may be more similar to the presentation of lower plexus compression. However, elbow flexion may commonly exacerbate these symptoms in cubital tunnel syndrome [10]. It must be noted, however that TOS may co-exist with these peripheral compressive neuropathies [11], so the positivity of these tests does not exclude a diagnosis of TOS.

Peripheral vascular examination should include palpation for a pulsatile mass in the supraclavicular and infraclavicular fossae, a sign of aneurysmal change. A bruit may also be auscultated [5]. Full status of the brachial, radial, and ulnar pulses should be recorded bilaterally. A blood pressure differential between arms of 20 mmHg may be found rarely in ATOS [25]. Whilst the above tests may not yield any findings in many cases of vascular TOS, provocative manoeuvres can be used to bring out these differences [2].

Commonly used provocative manoeuvres include EAST, ULTT, and Adson's test [2]. In the EAST, the scalene triangle is narrowed by abducting the arms to 90° with the elbows flexed, and the shoulder externally rotated slightly to tilt the forearms backwards. In this position, repetitive opening and closing of the fist may reproduce symptoms and lead to a reduction in radial pulse volume. The ULTT assesses recreation of symptoms from stretching the brachial plexus by holding the arm outstretched with the shoulder abducted to 90°, extension and the wrist and tilting the neck away from the limb being tested. Adson's test assesses for reproduction of symptoms or loss of radial pulse by extending the neck and rotating the head toward the symptomatic side whilst holding in deep inspiration. Provocative tests can add weight to a suspected diagnosis of TOS, but alone their utility is variable. One study found that 58% of random volunteers had at least one positive provocative test [26]. Indeed, when used alone, Adson's test and the EAST have specificity of 76% and 30%, respectively, but when the two provocative manoeuvres are used in conjunction, diagnostic specificity can rise to 82% [27].

4. Investigations

Investigations play two roles in TOS: (1) to confirm or add weight to the diagnosis of arterial, venous, or NTOS and (2) to suggest the anatomical cause of compression. A summary of the role that investigations play in the diagnosis of TOS can be found in Table 2. Once a diagnosis of TOS is suspected on clinical grounds, it is important to characterise the anatomy of the thoracic outlet, particularly with respect to potential sources of compression, as this can guide management approaches, especially if surgery is to be considered. Here, CT, chest radiography, and cervical spine films may show the presence of a cervical rib or elongated C7 transverse process. MRI on the other hand can evaluate soft tissue structures that might contribute to compression, such as fibrous bands, and can exclude cervical root compression as a differential diagnosis [28].

Table 2. Investigations in ATOS, VTOS, and NTOS.

TOS Subtype	Definite Role	Possible Role	Emerging Role
All	Plain radiography (chest/cervical spine) Non-contrast CT/MRI [5,27]	-	-
ATOS	Duplex ultrasound Contrast arteriography Finger plethysmography [5]	CT/MR arteriography with provocative manoeuvres [5,26,28–30]	-
VTOS	Duplex ultrasound [5,12,31] CT/MR venography [32] Contrast venography [33]	CT/MR venography with provocative manoeuvres [5,26,28]	-
NTOS	Nerve conduction studies Needle electromyography [5,34] Local anaesthetic injection test [5,35–38]	-	MR neurography [39,40] Diffusion tensor imaging [41–45] Brachial plexus ultrasound [46,47]

When it comes to supporting the suspected diagnosis, the mainstays of tests in ATOS are duplex ultrasound, arteriography, haemodynamic testing (e.g., finger plethysmography) at rest, and, with provocative manoeuvres, CT angiography and MR angiography [5]. Invasive arteriography and angiography are for detecting complications of ATOS such as thrombosis, embolisation, and aneurysm. Due to the invasive nature of these investigations, they are usually employed as part of surgery planning rather than diagnosis alone. More non-invasive tests such as MR and CT angiography have been studied for their use in diagnosis outside of the context of surgical planning. One benefit is that they can be used to dynamically evaluate arterial compression with provocative manoeuvres. Whilst there has been some controversy as to the utility of provocative testing for VTOS given that moderate to severe venous compression is common in healthy subjects, arterial compression is far less common [29]. However, studies show MR angiography cannot always distinguish between physiologic and pathologic compression, and the findings cannot always be correlated with clinical symptoms [30]. Recent evidence, however, has re-asserted the utility of dynamic CT angiography with the findings that significant subclavian artery stenosis on dynamic CT angiography is correlated with thoracic outlet symptomatology. In this recent study, patients with either unilateral or bilateral symptoms underwent CT angiography whilst in a supine position, with the arms in abduction of 120° and in external rotation, with the head turned toward the less pathological or asymptomatic side. Forty percent of symptomatic outlets, compared with 5% of asymptomatic outlets, had subclavian artery stenosis ≥50% [31]. These findings in dynamic CT angiography are encouraging; however, while these investigations may lend weight toward a diagnosis of ATOS, a diagnosis cannot be made on these findings in isolation. The overall clinical picture, in the absence of detection of a thrombus, embolus, or aneurysm, therefore becomes paramount.

In diagnosing VTOS, duplex ultrasound is typically employed if thrombosis is suspected, with very high sensitivity and specificity of 78–100% and 82–100%, respectively. However, its use in cases without thrombosis is equivocal [12,32]. Even in the context of venous thrombosis, there are limitations to the use of ultrasound such as the shadow cast by the overlying clavicle over the proximal subclavian vein. In this situation, CT and MR venography can be used to demonstrate the extent of the thrombus, the degree of collateralisation, the point of compression, and the associated anatomical abnormalities [33]. If intervention is to be planned, such as catheter-directed thrombolysis or percutaneous transluminal angioplasty, contrast venography is the gold standard [34]. However, in the absence of thrombosis, imaging even with provocative manoeuvres will not be diagnostic on its own [29].

NTOS is a field where the contribution of diagnostic investigations is certainly changing. In cases of suspected TOS presumed not to be secondary to venous or arterial compression, classically electrodiagnostic studies were used to stratify cases of "true" NTOS from "disputed" NTOS—cases of similar symptomatology but lacking such conduction defects. However, given the fact that conduction defects may not be apparent at earlier stages, this distinction is being phased out [5]. Recently, however, there is suggestion that conduction deficits are present in a much larger group of patients with NTOS. Tsao et al. found that, upon testing the medial antebrachial cutaneous nerve and median motor nerve supplying the abductor pollicis brevis, T1 and C8 derived fibres commonly show conduction deficits. When electrodiagnostics combined medial antebrachial cutaneous nerve with median motor nerve testing, findings were abnormal in 89% of patients with NTOS [35]. This suggests that electrodiagnostic tests can still be used to support a diagnosis of TOS, even in its early stages.

Another testing modality suggested by the Society for Vascular Surgery is to inject the scalene and pectoralis minor muscles with local anaesthetic to check for alleviation of symptoms, the rationale being that the scalene triangle and pectoralis minor space are common sites of compression [5]. As alleviation of symptoms will only occur if the injected muscle is the source of compression, rather than a fibrous band for example, this also acts as a localisation test. Although this technique has been around for a while, having first been proposed by Gage in 1939 [36], it is still being adapted, such as the technique for the use of ultrasound guided anterior scalene and pectoralis minor blocks in high-performance overhead athletes who may often have subtle examination findings. In these patients, studying symptomatic changes while such patients exercise may be advisable [37]. Furthermore, it is only relatively recently that the degree of symptomatic and functional improvement has been fully characterised. Braun et al. [38] assessed the use of scalene blocks in individuals with symptomatology suggesting a diagnosis of thoracic outlet syndrome. Electrodiagnostics, imaging, and orthopaedic opinion were used to rule out differential diagnoses. Fingertip sensation was tested before and after the block to rule out changes secondary to sensory plexus nerve block. Compared with sternocleidomastoid injection controls, all patients with anterior scalene muscle blocks noted symptomatic and functional improvement after the blocks, with an increase in their work capacity in waist level push–pull tests by 93%, overhead bar push–pull tests by 108%, and extremity abduction stress test with repetitive hand gripping during static arm elevation by 104%. Time to fatigue and power also increased after the block. The hope is that by quantifying these parameters, diagnostically significant improvements in symptoms and function post-block can be more objectively assessed. Scalene blocks also appear to be prognostic in certain groups when it comes to predicting surgical outcome. In one study, lidocaine rather than botulinum toxin blocks were predictive of better outcomes in patients following transaxillary decompression. These were more noticeable in patients ≥40 years (14% improvement in surgical success) compared with patients <40 years (7% improvement), perhaps due to the fact that younger patients generally tend to have better surgical outcomes than older patients [39].

Increasingly it is being realised that MRI can be used not only to evaluate the anatomy of the thoracic outlet, in particular soft tissue structures that might be causing compression, but also to visualise actual compression of the brachial plexus directly. With the use of high-resolution MRI scanners with a 3.0 T magnetic field strength, MR neurography (MRN) allows nerve morphology and signal to be non-invasively visualised. This technique suppresses signal from surrounding soft tissue structures, including fat containing structures, and removes pulsation artefacts from flowing blood [40]. In this way, the exact site of compression as well as the structure causing the compression can be identified directly, instead of having to indirectly infer that the presence of a fibrous band may be the cause of compression in a patient with documented NTOS. Baumer et al. used high-resolution MRN in patients with suspicion of neurogenic or non-specified TOS to identify cases brachial plexus compression. All cases identified were subsequently verified by surgical exploration, showing good positive predictive value of this investigation. This study, however, did not verify by surgical exploration those without discernible defects on MRN, so the negative predictive value of this test is not known [41].

MRI can be applied in another modality: that of diffusion tensor imaging (DTI). This technique works on the principle of the non-random and distinct movement of water molecules through highly organised cell structures of myelinated nerve bundles [40]. Evidence suggests that the quantitative parameters generated with DTI (fractional anisotropy and axial, radial, and mean diffusivity) may correlate with the mechanism of neuropathy. One study found that, by correlating DTI findings with electrophysiology in an assessment of the median nerve in the carpal tunnel, axial diffusivity reflected axon integrity, whereas radial diffusivity and functional anisotropy reflected myelin sheath integrity [42]. Indeed, this technique has shown promise in other peripheral neuropathies including carpal tunnel syndrome. One study performed DTI on the median nerve in subjects with carpal tunnel syndrome and compared with control subjects and showed that the measured parameters in DTI show a highly significant difference ($p < 0.0001$) [43]. The reproducibility of findings, as well as the intra- and inter-evaluator agreement when it comes to the application of DTI to the brachia plexus, however, does have good evidence [44], with one study estimating reproducibility of 81–92% when healthy volunteers were imaged [45]. Although application of this technology to NTOS has not yet been reflected in the literature, there is evidence for the use of DTI in other brachial plexus injuries. One feasibility study aimed to use DTI at 1.5 T to detect nerve root avulsions in patients with brachial plexus injuries and found it to have an overall accuracy of 94.5%, including detection of both complete and partial avulsions [46].

Ultrasound imaging, a staple in VTOS, may also be applied to NTOS, with the benefit over MRI being the low cost and more readily available nature of the technology. Leonhard et al. demonstrated that there is a significant increase in the incidence of symptoms of NTOS in patients with brachial plexus variants in which portions of the proximal plexus pierce the anterior scalene and thereby may be susceptible to impingement within the muscle belly. These branching variants can be identified by ultrasonography. Of 22 subjects, 21% demonstrated this atypical branching anatomy on ultrasonography. Fifty percent of these subjects reported symptoms consistent with NTOS, versus 14% in those with classical brachial plexus anatomy [47]. Knowledge of the branching anatomy of the brachial plexus can be used to guide management, including surgery and may be used in future trials that stratify treatment approaches based on the branching anatomy. It has also been suggested that ultrasonography of the thoracic outlet can be used to dynamically evaluate brachial plexus compression, which would be highly suitable in the outpatient setting. In this technique, when an ultrasound probe is placed in the supraclavicular fossa, the brachial plexus can be visualised generally above and just posterior to the subclavian artery, and can be seen in relation to the surrounding anterior and middle scalene muscles. When the patient is asked to abduct the arm in performance of the EAST, reduction in the interscalene interval, compression of the brachial plexus, or obliteration of the visualised nerves can be correlated with the reproduction of symptoms to add weight to a diagnosis of NTOS [48]. This technique, however, requires more rigorous evaluation.

5. Summary and Perspective

As we can see, diagnosis of TOS is complicated by the variety of presentations, the number of differential diagnoses, including co-existence of diagnoses such as arterial with NTOS and peripheral compressive neuropathies with TOS, and the variable reliability of provocative manoeuvres and investigations when used in isolation. In this context, the diagnosis requires high-quality clinical acumen with respect to history taking and examination, with investigations often used more to add weight to a suspected diagnosis. As discussed, imaging is used to evaluate the anatomy of the thoracic outlet to guide management, such as whether to excise a cervical rib. However, in the absence of such abnormalities, the exact mechanism of compression may not be fully understood. It is therefore encouraging to see ongoing developments in this area, including dynamic CT angiography, MR neurography, DTI, and the use of ultrasound, including an article recently published in this journal, which showed that it can be used to identify brachial plexus branching variants in which susceptibility to compression by the scalene muscle is increased [47]. Developments of similar tools may begin to stratify patients according to the pathophysiology of compression, rather than purely on their respective clusters of symptoms, may pave the way in developing more specific treatments.

Conflicts of Interest: The authors declare no conflict of interest.

References

1. Peet, R.M.; Henriksen, J.D.; Anderson, T.P.; Martin, G.M. Thoracic-outlet syndrome: Evaluation of a therapeutic exercise program. *Proc. Staff Meet. Mayo Clin.* **1956**, *31*, 281–287. [PubMed]
2. Kuhn, J.E.; Lebus, V.G.F.; Bible, J.E. Thoracic outlet syndrome. *J. Am. Acad. Orthop. Surg.* **2015**, *23*, 222–232. [CrossRef] [PubMed]
3. Klaassen, Z.; Sorenson, E.; Tubbs, R.S.; Arya, R.; Meloy, P.; Shah, R.; Shirk, S.; Loukas, M. Thoracic outlet syndrome: A neurological and vascular disorder. *Clin. Anat.* **2014**, *27*, 724–732. [CrossRef] [PubMed]
4. Ozoa, G.; Alves, D.; Fish, D.E. Thoracic outlet syndrome. *Phys. Med. Rehabil. Clin. N. Am.* **2011**, *22*, 473–483. [CrossRef] [PubMed]
5. Illig, K.A.; Donahue, D.; Duncan, A.; Freischlag, J.; Gelabert, H.; Johansen, K.; Jordan, S.; Sanders, R.; Thompson, R. Reporting standards of the society for vascular surgery for thoracic outlet syndrome. *J. Vasc. Surg.* **2016**, *64*, 23–35. [CrossRef] [PubMed]
6. Povlsen, B.; Hansson, T.; Povlsen, S.D. Treatment for thoracic outlet syndrome. *Cochrane Database Syst. Rev.* **2014**. [CrossRef] [PubMed]
7. Sanders, R.J.; Hammond, S.L.; Rao, N.M. Diagnosis of thoracic outlet syndrome. *J. Vasc. Surg.* **2007**, *46*, 601–604. [CrossRef] [PubMed]
8. Woods, B.I.; Hilibrand, A.S. Cervical radiculopathy: Epidemiology, etiology, diagnosis, and treatment. *Clin. Spine Surg.* **2015**, *28*, E251–E259. [CrossRef] [PubMed]
9. Middleton, S.D.; Anakwe, R.E. Carpal tunnel syndrome. *Br. Med. J.* **2014**. [CrossRef] [PubMed]
10. Kroonen, L.T. Cubital tunnel syndrome. *Orthop. Clin. N. Am.* **2012**, *43*, 475–486. [CrossRef] [PubMed]
11. Hooper, T.L.; Denton, J.; McGalliard, M.K.; Brismée, J.M.; Sizer, P.S. Thoracic outlet syndrome: A controversial clinical condition. Part 1: Anatomy, and clinical examination/diagnosis. *J. Man. Manip. Ther.* **2010**, *18*, 74–83. [CrossRef] [PubMed]
12. Moore, R.; Lum, Y.W. Venous thoracic outlet syndrome. *Vasc. Med.* **2015**, *20*, 182–189. [CrossRef] [PubMed]
13. Shutze, W.; Richardson, B.; Shutze, R.; Tran, K.; Dao, A.; Ogola, G.O.; Young, A.; Pearl, G. Midterm and long-term follow-up in competitive athletes undergoing thoracic outlet decompression for neurogenic thoracic outlet syndrome. *J. Vasc. Surg.* **2017**, *66*, 1798–1805. [CrossRef] [PubMed]
14. Duwayri, Y.M.; Emery, V.B.; Driskill, M.R.; Earley, J.A.; Wright, R.W.; Paletta, G.A.; Thompson, R.W. Positional compression of the axillary artery causing upper extremity thrombosis and embolism in the elite overhead throwing athlete. *J. Vasc. Surg.* **2011**, *53*, 1329–1340. [CrossRef] [PubMed]
15. Campbell, R.M. Thoracic outlet syndrome in musicians—An approach to treatment. *Work* **1996**, *7*, 115–119. [CrossRef]
16. Adam, G.; Wang, K.; Demaree, C.J.; Jiang, J.S.; Cheung, M.; Bechara, C.F.; Lin, P.H. A prospective evaluation of duplex ultrasound for thoracic outlet syndrome in high-performance musicians playing bowed string instruments. *Diagnostics* **2018**, *8*, 11. [CrossRef] [PubMed]
17. Gilliatt, R.W.; Le Quesne, P.M.; Logue, V.; Sumner, A.J. Wasting of the hand associated with a cervical rib or band. *J. Neurol. Neurosurg. Psychiatry* **1970**, *33*, 615–624. [CrossRef] [PubMed]
18. Diercks, R.; Bron, C.; Dorrestijn, O.; Meskers, C.; Naber, R.; de Ruiter, T.; Willems, J.; Winters, J.; van der Woude, H.J. Guideline for diagnosis and treatment of subacromial pain syndrome: A multidisciplinary review by the Dutch Orthopaedic Association. *Acta Orthop.* **2014**, *85*, 314–322. [CrossRef] [PubMed]
19. Neviaser, A.S.; Neviaser, R.J. Adhesive capsulitis of the shoulder. *J. Am. Acad. Orthop. Surg.* **2011**, *19*, 536–542. [CrossRef] [PubMed]
20. Eljabu, W.; Klinger, H.M.; von Knoch, M. The natural history of rotator cuff tears: A systematic review. *Arch. Orthop. Trauma Surg.* **2015**, *135*, 1055–1061. [CrossRef] [PubMed]
21. Jain, N.B.; Luz, J.; Higgins, L.D.; Dong, Y.; Warner, J.J.; Matzkin, E.; Katz, J.N. The diagnostic accuracy of special tests for rotator cuff tear: The ROW cohort study. *Am. J. Phys. Med. Rehabil.* **2017**, *96*, 176–183. [CrossRef] [PubMed]

22. Thatte, M.R.; Babhulkar, S.; Hiremath, A. Brachial plexus injury in adults: Diagnosis and surgical treatment strategies. *Ann. Indian Acad. Neurol.* **2013**, *16*, 26–33. [CrossRef] [PubMed]
23. Atasoy, E. A hand surgeon's further experience with thoracic outlet compression syndrome. *J. Hand Surg.* **2010**, *35*, 1528–1538. [CrossRef] [PubMed]
24. Bruske, J.; Bednarski, M.; Grzelec, H.; Zyluk, A. The usefulness of the Phalen test and the Hoffmann-Tinel sign in the diagnosis of carpal tunnel syndrome. *Acta Orthop. Belg.* **2002**, *68*, 141–145. [PubMed]
25. Brantigan, C.O.; Roos, D.B. Diagnosing thoracic outlet syndrome. *Hand Clin.* **2004**, *20*, 27–36. [CrossRef]
26. Warrens, A.N.; Heaton, J.M. Thoracic outlet compression syndrome: The lack of reliability of its clinical assessment. *Ann. R. Coll. Surg. Engl.* **1987**, *69*, 203–204. [PubMed]
27. Gillard, J.; Pérez-Cousin, M.; Hachulla, É.; Remy, J.; Hurtevent, J.F.; Vinckier, L.; Thévenon, A.; Duquesnoy, B. Diagnosing thoracic outlet syndrome: Contribution of provocative tests, ultrasonography, electrophysiology, and helical computed tomography in 48 patients. *Jt. Bone Spine* **2001**, *68*, 416–424. [CrossRef]
28. Kuwayama, D.P.; Lund, J.R.; Brantigan, C.O.; Glebova, N.O. Choosing surgery for neurogenic TOS: The roles of physical exam, physical therapy, and imaging. *Diagnostics* **2017**, *7*, 37. [CrossRef] [PubMed]
29. Matsumura, J.S.; Rilling, W.S.; Pearce, W.H.; Nemcek, A.A.; Vogelzang, R.L.; Yao, J.S. Helical computed tomography of the normal thoracic outlet. *J. Vasc. Surg.* **1997**, *26*, 776–783. [CrossRef]
30. Aralasmak, A.; Cevikol, C.; Karaali, K.; Senol, U.; Sharifov, R.; Kilicarslan, R.; Alkan, A. MRI findings in thoracic outlet syndrome. *Skelet. Radiol.* **2012**, *41*, 1365–1374. [CrossRef] [PubMed]
31. Gillet, R.; Teixeira, P.; Meyer, J.B.; Rauch, A.; Raymond, A.; Dap, F.; Blum, A. Dynamic CT angiography for the diagnosis of patients with thoracic outlet syndrome: Correlation with patient symptoms. *J. Cardiovasc. Comput. Tomogr.* **2017**. [CrossRef] [PubMed]
32. Butros, S.R.; Liu, R.; Oliveira, G.R.; Ganguli, S.; Kalva, S. Venous compression syndromes: Clinical features, imaging findings and management. *Br. J. Radiol.* **2013**, *86*, 20130284. [CrossRef] [PubMed]
33. Demondion, X.; Herbinet, P.; Van Sint Jan, S.; Boutry, N.; Chantelot, C.; Cotten, A. Imaging assessment of thoracic outlet syndrome. *Radiographics* **2006**, *26*, 1735–1750. [CrossRef] [PubMed]
34. Landry, G.J.; Liem, T.K. Endovascular management of Paget-Schroetter syndrome. *Vascular* **2007**, *15*, 290–296. [CrossRef] [PubMed]
35. Tsao, B.E.; Ferrante, M.A.; Wilbourn, A.J.; Shields, R.W. Electrodiagnostic features of true neurogenic thoracic outlet syndrome. *Muscle Nerve* **2014**, *49*, 724–727. [CrossRef] [PubMed]
36. Gage, M. Scalenus anticus syndrome: A diagnostic and confirmatory test. *Surgery* **1939**, *5*, 599–601. [CrossRef]
37. Bottros, M.M.; AuBuchon, J.D.; McLaughlin, L.N.; Altchek, D.W.; Illig, K.A.; Thompson, R.W. Exercise-enhanced, ultrasound-guided anterior scalene muscle/pectoralis minor muscle blocks can facilitate the diagnosis of neurogenic thoracic outlet syndrome in the high-performance overhead athlete. *Am. J. Sports Med.* **2017**, *45*, 189–194. [CrossRef] [PubMed]
38. Braun, R.M.; Shah, K.N.; Rechnic, M.; Doehr, S.; Woods, N. Quantitative assessment of scalene muscle block for the diagnosis of suspected thoracic outlet syndrome. *J. Hand Surg. Am.* **2015**, *40*, 2255–2261. [CrossRef] [PubMed]
39. Lum, Y.W.; Brooke, B.S.; Likes, K.; Modi, M.; Grunebach, H.; Christo, P.J.; Freischlag, J.A. Impact of anterior scalene lidocaine blocks on predicting surgical success in older patients with neurogenic thoracic outlet syndrome. *J. Vasc. Surg.* **2012**, *55*, 1370–1375. [CrossRef] [PubMed]
40. Magill, S.T.; Brus-Ramer, M.; Weinstein, P.R.; Chin, C.T.; Jacques, L. Neurogenic thoracic outlet syndrome: Current diagnostic criteria and advances in MRI diagnostics. *Neurosurg. Focus* **2015**, *39*, E7. [CrossRef] [PubMed]
41. Baumer, P.; Kele, H.; Kretschmer, T.; Koenig, R.; Pedro, M.; Bendszus, M.; Pham, M. Thoracic outlet syndrome in 3T MR neurography-fibrous bands causing discernible lesions of the lower brachial plexus. *Eur. Radiol.* **2014**, *24*, 756–761. [CrossRef] [PubMed]
42. Heckel, A.; Weiler, M.; Xia, A.; Ruetters, M.; Pham, M.; Bendszus, M.; Heiland, S.; Baeumer, P. Peripheral nerve diffusion tensor imaging: Assessment of axon and myelin sheath integrity. *PLoS ONE* **2015**, *10*, e0130833. [CrossRef] [PubMed]
43. Stein, D.; Neufeld, A.; Pasternak, O.; Graif, M.; Patish, H.; Schwimmer, E.; Ziv, E.; Assaf, Y. Diffusion tensor imaging of the median nerve in healthy and carpal tunnel syndrome subjects. *J. Magn. Reson. Imaging* **2009**, *29*, 657–662. [CrossRef] [PubMed]

44. Ho, M.J.; Manoliu, A.; Kuhn, F.P.; Stieltjes, B.; Klarhöfer, M.; Feiweier, T.; Marcon, M.; Andreisek, G. Evaluation of reproducibility of diffusion tensor imaging in the brachial plexus at 3.0 T. *Investig. Radiol.* **2017**, *52*, 482–487. [CrossRef] [PubMed]

45. Tagliafico, A.; Calabrese, M.; Puntoni, M.; Pace, D.; Baio, G.; Neumaier, C.E.; Martinoli, C. Brachial plexus MR imaging: Accuracy and reproducibility of DTI-derived measurements and fibre tractography at 3.0-T. *Eur. Radiol.* **2011**, *21*, 1764–1771. [CrossRef] [PubMed]

46. Gasparotti, R.; Lodoli, G.; Meoded, A.; Carletti, F.; Garozzo, D.; Ferraresi, S. Feasibility of diffusion tensor tractography of brachial plexus injuries at 1.5 T. *Investig. Radiol.* **2013**, *48*, 104–112. [CrossRef] [PubMed]

47. Leonhard, V.; Caldwell, G.; Goh, M.; Reeder, S.; Smith, H.F. Ultrasonographic diagnosis of thoracic outlet syndrome secondary to brachial plexus piercing variation. *Diagnostics* **2017**, *7*, 40. [CrossRef] [PubMed]

48. Fried, S.M.; Nazarian, L.N. Dynamic neuromusculoskeletal ultrasound documentation of brachial plexus/thoracic outlet compression during elevated arm stress testing. *Hand* **2013**, *8*, 358–365. [CrossRef] [PubMed]

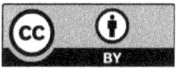

MDPI

St. Alban-Anlage 66

4052 Basel

Switzerland

Tel. +41 61 683 77 34

Fax +41 61 302 89 18

www.mdpi.com

Diagnostics Editorial Office

E-mail: diagnostics@mdpi.com

www.mdpi.com/journal/diagnostics

www.ingramcontent.com/pod-product-compliance
Lightning Source LLC
Chambersburg PA
CBHW051914210326
41597CB00033B/6145